GW00949792

A System of Hypnotherapy

A System of Hypnotherapy

B. J. Hartman

Nelson-Hall nh Chicago

Library of Congress Cataloging in Publication Data

Hartman, Bernard James.
  A system of hypnotherapy.

  Bibliography: p.
  Includes index.
  1. Hypnotism—Therapeutic use. I. Title.
RC495.H38   615'.8512   79-16980
ISBN 0-88229-449-0

Copyright © 1980 by Bernard J. Hartman

Manufactured in the United States of America

10   9   8   7   6   5   4   3   2   1

Contents

Part Seven
Research and Training
in Hypnotherapy

Foreword

We doctors are often assumed to know how to do all procedures, but we frequently find that these assumptions are wrong. In my own practice I have a constant need for a reference encompassing instructions and some guidelines and even something that will give me some fresh thoughts. Over a period of years I have learned to rely upon compiled books and notes.

A System of Hypnotherapy, by Dr. B. J. Hartman is a unique book in that it provides a system of structured learning. An excellent one for reference, an equally excellent one as a text. *A System Of Hypnotherapy* is a step-by-step structured learning procedure taking you carefully through the high points of theory, into induction, the stages of hypnosis, the types of hypnosis and the advantages of using various types such as hypnoidal, direct, analysis and reconstruction. Dr. Hartman even takes you into the hypnotic treatment, including references to narco hypnoanalysis as well. His references, research material and training are all outlined clearly and succinctly. His references are broad and of excellent material. At the close of the book, he has included a glossary for those who may be in need. I have found it to be an excellent one.

This book, in my opinion, should be in everyone's library. The step-by-step structured learning method as outlined and discussed in detail in *A System of Hypnotherapy* is recommended to you without equivocation. It is my sincere wish that you will find it as interesting as I have and that this volume will be helpful in your day-to-day practice.

James L. Rowland, M.S., D.O., Ph.D., F.A.C.G.P., Past President, International Society for Professional Hypnosis

Preface

I have entitled this book *A System of Hypnotherapy* because my purpose has been to describe hypnotherapy as I practice it. I have long felt the need for an all-inclusive and eclectic system of hypnotherapy that has a clear rationale with specific indications and contraindications for each type of therapy as well as specific techniques to be used within each approach. In this way, hypnotherapy can be appreciated as a system of treatment in which various approaches are linked together by their clear relation to underlying psychodynamic theory.

The system of hypnotherapy to be described is an outgrowth of personal experience with many types of clients over the past fourteen years and represents an integration and synthesis of the various approaches to hypnotherapy existent in the literature. Although a great deal of clinical research has preceded the development of my system of hypnotherapy in its present form, I view it as something dynamic, flexible and in need of constant refinement in light of findings from ongoing clinical research.

This book differs from all others that have been published in the area of hypnotherapy in two very important respects. One is the system of hypnotherapy itself. This is the first book in the field to present a systematic approach to hypnotherapy with specific types, specific techniques for each type and specific phases of hypnotherapy. The other unique aspect of this book is the structured learning approach to training, which has four essential components: modeling of the desired skill, role playing of the desired skill by the trainees, immediate feedback and transfer of training in the form of specific homework assignments. This step-by-step approach to training has proven to be highly effective in training hypnotherapists.

Much of the material in this book has been presented to hundreds of psychologists, psychiatric social workers, psychiatrists, psychology interns and psychiatric residents in classes that I have taught on hypnotherapy and hypnoanalysis. I want to thank them for their feedback regarding the use of the system of hypnotherapy presented in this book with a wide variety of clients.

Acknowledgments

The author wishes to thank his wife, Claire, for numerous hours spent in typing the manuscript and to acknowledge courtesies extended him by the following publications from which papers have been reprinted wholly or in part:

Hypnosis Research and Practice

> Hartman, B. J.   Special techniques of hypnoanalysis. 1968, **1**, (2), 4-10.

> Hartman, B. J.   Accidental autohypnosis: a hypnocybernetic approach to emotional disorders. 1969, **2**, (2), 8-13.

> Hartman, B. J.   The treatment of disorders of sexual function by hypnotherapy. 1970, **3**, (2), 7-10.

> Hartman, B. J.   The treatment of menstrual disorders by hypnotherapy. 1971, **4**, (1), 17-20.

Journal of the National Medical Association

> Hartman, B. J.   The use of hypnosis in the treatment of drug addiction. 1972, **64**, (1), 35-38.

> Hartman, B. J.   Hypnotherapeutic approaches to the treatment of alcoholism. 1976, **68**, 101-103.

Journal of the International Society for Professional Hypnosis

> Hartman, B. J.   The use of hypnodrama in assertive training. 1973, **2**, (4), 15-18.

> Hartman, B. J.   The use of hypnosis in the treatment of the Rip Van Winkle syndrome. 1975, **4**, (2), 31-34.

American Journal of Clinical Hypnosis

> Hartman, B. J.   Group hypnotherapy in a university counseling center. 1969, **12**, 16-19.

Part One
Theoretical and
Phenomenological
Aspects of Hypnosis

Chapter 1.

Theories of Hypnosis

No theory adequately explains all the phenomena of hypnosis. It is likely that when we know more about the mind, a comprehensive theory incorporating various aspects of the many existing theories will be developed.

Theories of hypnosis fall into two major categories: the physiological ones, which view hypnosis as an altered condition of the brain, and the psychological ones, which view it as a unique interpersonal relationship. Some theories attempt to combine the two points of view. Theories are classified according to the kind of manifestations they interpret hypnosis to be.

HYPNOSIS AS A NEUROPHYSIOLOGICAL MANIFESTATION

Many theorists contend that hypnosis is due to a changed physiology of the cerebral cortex. Heidenhain (1906) believed in an inhibition of the ganglion cells of the brain. Wolberg (1948) believed that the spreading of inhibition over higher cortical centers is a partial explanation of hypnosis. Young (1941) contended that hypnosis is due to the inhibition of one set of mental functions and excitation of others. McDougall (1926) held that hypnosis is caused by a shift of nervous energies of the central nervous system to the vasomotor system. Kubie and Margolin (1944) contended that hypnosis is due to a focus of central excitation with surrounding areas of inhibition. Estabrooks (1943) suggested that hypnosis is

3

due to synaptic ablation, whereby neural impulses are directed into a smaller number of channels. Pavlov (1957) held that hypnosis is due to a radiation of cerebral inhibition following repeated and monotonous stimulation. Bartlett (1968) postulated a theory on the action mechanism of hypnosis as an increasing integration of the neocortex and the subcortical areas of the brain, with the subcortical areas activated to a greater extent than normally.

Roberts (1960, 1963) contended that interruption between the brain stem reticular formation and the specific sensory, parasensory and coordinated neuronal channels results in hypnosis.

> It is proposed that hypnotic trance may be correlated physiologically with an induced hyperpolarization of the deep pyramidal cells of the cerebral cortex in a waking subject. An activation of the reticulo-unspecific system of the brain, simultaneous with a disactivation of specific corticopetal pathways, during hypnotic induction, is assumed to be the cause of a marked inhibitory change in cortical electrotonus. The unspecific activation and the specific disactivation may represent the physiological counterparts of hypnotic "fixation" and the hypnogenic "reduction of afferent input," respectively. [Roberts, 1963, pp. 9-10]

HYPNOSIS AS A CONDITIONED RESPONSE

This theory is held by a number of contemporary investigators, including Jacobson (1938), Salter (1944), Eysenck (1947), Wolpe (1958) and Korth (1958). Pavlov (1957), Hull (1933) and Young (1941) were also proponents of words as conditioned stimuli, Salter, the leading proponent of this theory, stated:

> Hypnosis basically involves conditioned reactions and reflexes. Some people have conditionings which we can evoke to create the so-called "trance" state. In this state it is possible to give verbalisms of behavior to be carried out on the occurrence of an after-awakening "bell"—so-called post-hypnotic suggestion. [1944, p. 8]

HYPNOSIS AS A PATHOLOGICAL MANIFESTATION

Charcot (1889), Binet and Fere (1888) and Janet (1920) considered hypnosis to be a symptom of hysteria. The formulations leading to this theoretical conclusion were based upon a small number of mental hospital patients. This theory was discredited by the fact that normal individuals are readily hypnotizable.

HYPNOSIS AS A STATE OF IMMOBILIZATION

This theory compares hypnosis with the tonic immobilization in animals. Tonic immobilization is produced primarily by physical and instinctual factors and results from these factors interacting with the symbolic meaning of words. Pavlov (1957), Meares (1960) and Schneck (1953) can be included here.

HYPNOSIS AS SLEEP OR A SLEEPLIKE STATE

Older investigators considered hypnosis a modified form of sleep. Modern research has demonstrated that hypnosis has the physiological indices of the conscious state. Pavlov (1957) was the major proponent of this theory. Despite the fact that all of the research has been to the contrary, there are still at least two modern proponents of this theory—Weber (1956) and Sparks (1960).

HYPNOSIS AS A STATE OF DISSOCIATION

Janet (1920), Prince (1929), Sidis (1910) and Burnett (1925) employed this explanation. Hypnosis was believed to abolish volition and leave only a reflexlike type of behavior, which was dissociated from consciousness. This theory was discredited when it was demonstrated that there was hyperacuity of all of the senses during hypnosis, that amnesia could be removed by suggestions of the hypnotic operator and that amnesia would not always occur spontaneously.

HYPNOSIS AS A STATE OF HYPERSUGGESTIBILITY

Although most investigators hold hypnosis to be a state of increased suggestibility, there are opponents even of this view. Brown (1919), for example, has stated that suggestibility decreases in deep hypnosis.

HYPNOSIS AS A PSYCHOSOMATIC MANIFESTATION

A number of investigators regard hypnosis as being both physiological and psychological in character. Wolberg (1948) held that hypnotic phenomena are due to a psychosomatic reaction consisting of a reciprocal and dynamic interaction of physiological and psychological factors. From the physiological standpoint, Wolberg contended that hypnosis is a spreading of inhibition over the higher centers in the cortex. On the psychological side, he believed hypnosis to be a transference phenomenon.

Kubie and Margolin (1944) also held a psychosomatic viewpoint. They proposed that hypnosis involves an extension of the subject's own psychic processes so as to include the voice of the hypnotic operator.

Weitzenhoffer (1953) theorized that suggestibility and hypnotic phenomena have a multiple origin based on psychosomatic processes. Weitzenhoffer contended that the voice of the hypnotic operator becomes an extension of the hypnotic subject's psychic processes, resulting in a large variety of perceptual alterations.

Hypnosis as a Goal-directed Striving

White (1941) was the first to clearly express the view that the subject attempts to behave like a hypnotized person as defined by the hypnotic operator and understood by the subject. The hypnotic subject, according to White, understands at all times what the operator intends, and his behavior strives to put these intentions into execution. McDougall (1926), Rosenow (1928), Lundholm (1928), Pattie (1937), Dorcus (1937) and Schilder and Kauders (1956) are additional advocates of this theory.

Hypnosis as Role Taking

Sarbin (1950, 1963) contended that hypnosis is a form of general social-psychological behavior that he calls role taking: the hypnotic subject strives to take the role of the hypnotized person. According to Sarbin, hypnosis is only a word for a special type of culturally defined influence situation, and there is no need to postulate a special state or trance.

In Sarbin's theory, the similarity between role taking in drama and in hypnosis is noted. Sarbin contended that a common denominator is operative in both forms of conduct and that success in the achievement of either role depends upon at least three attributes: (1) the accuracy of the actor's perception of the role demands; (2) the motivation to perform; and (3) skill or aptitude in role enactment.

Hypnosis as a Habit Phenomenon

Hull (1933) based his theory of hypnosis primarily on two interrelated postulates: (1) hypnotic suggestibility is a habit phenomenon; and (2) the most important characteristic of a habit phenomenon is that it is facilitated by practice.

IDEOMOTOR ACTIVITY AND INHIBITION THEORY

Some theorists contend that the effects of suggestibility are the result of ideomotor action and inhibition, and that suggestibility is merely an experience of imagining that which is actualized through ideomotor activities. Arnold (1946) and Eysenck (1947) are advocates of this theory. This time-worn theory, originally presented by William James, explains automatic movements that are induced, but it gives no adequate explanation for the highly complicated psychological reactions characteristic of the hypnotic state.

THE ANIMAL MAGNETISM THEORY

This was the earliest theory to receive serious attention by hypnotic investigators. Mesmer (1948) held that hypnosis or mesmerism was due to a magnetic force called animal magnetism, which emanated from the body of the hypnotizer and affected the subject. Although animal magnetism was discredited even in Mesmer's time, it still has a few modern exponents who believe that a human magnetic force is the cause of hypnosis.

SUPERCONCENTRATION OF THE MIND THEORY

Van Pelt (1958) believed that hypnosis is a superconcentration of the mind, a concentrating of the various mental activities into a single ray. Van Pelt stated:

> In the ordinary state the mind is occupied with many different impressions, so that mind power is scattered. . . . In hypnosis the mind is concentrated to a degree much higher than possible in the ordinary state. Practically all the suggestion is absorbed, and so the effect is strong. [1958, p. 4]

HYPNOSIS AS A BYPASSING OF THE CRITICAL FACULTY

Elman (1964) held that hypnosis is simply a state of mind in which that part of the mind which passes judgment is bypassed and in which an idea is accepted wholeheartedly.

ATAVISTIC THEORIES

Kroger and Freed (1956) held that hypnotic behavior is an atavism that at one time may have been necessary in humans as a protective defense mechanism to ward off fear or danger. Meares (1960) also held an atavistic hypothesis, stating that hypnosis is a return to a more primitive form of mental functioning in which suggestion plays a major role.

Psychokinetic Theory of Hypnosis

Muftic (1959) contended that hypnosis is due to psychokinetic field forces involving cortical areas through extrasensory perceptions in a manner similar to oscillating electromagnetic fields.

Psychoanalytic Theories of Hypnosis

Psychoanalytic theories of hypnosis are based on the premise that instinctual wishes of the hypnotic subject are elicited and given some gratification by the hypnotic situation. A number of psychoanalytically oriented theorists, including Ferenczi (1916), Jones (1913), Lorand (1941) and Kubie and Margolin (1944) viewed hypnosis as a form of transference, meaning that the hypnotic subject acts under the dominance of unconscious, infantile, instinctual drives.

Ferenczi (1916) held that hypnosis is a regression to infancy in which the hypnotic operator assumes the role of the parent. He differentiated maternal and paternal forms of hypnosis, maternal based on love and paternal based on fear.

Freud (1922) compared hypnosis to being in love. He stated:

> There is the same humble subjection, the same compliance, the same absence of criticism toward the hypnotist just as toward the loved object . . . The hypnotic relation is the devotion of someone in love to an unlimited degree but with sexual satisfaction excluded. [p. 77]

Jones (1923) stressed narcissism in his paper on autosuggestion.

> Suggestion is essentially a libidinal process; through the unification of the various forms and derivatives of narcissism the criticizing faculty of the ego-ideal is suspended so that ego-syntonic ideas are able to follow unchecked the pleasure-pain principle in accordance with a primitive belief in the omnipotence of thought. [1923, p. 206]

Ego-psychological Theory

Bellak (1955) perceived hypnosis as being a special type of self-excluding function of the ego. A change occurs from conscious perception to preconscious functioning and this is regarded as a topological regression, he theorized.

Metapsychological Theory of Hypnosis

Gill and Brenman (1959) regarded hypnosis as a regression in the service of the ego. Their metapsychological treatment of hypnosis as a regression rests on the concept of relative autonomy of the ego from the id, the concept of relative autonomy of the ego from the environment, and the relationship between these two autonomies. Gill and Brenman stated:

> Hypnosis is a condition of loss of autonomy with domination of a subsystem of the ego by a part of the social environment. Hypnosis is characterized by the fact that the subject is in a regressed state and engages in regressive interpersonal relationships. Hypnosis is therefore both an altered state and a transference relationship. The normal ego maintains relative autonomy from drives within and the environment from without. [1959, p. 195]

Harmony Theory

Teitelbaum (1965) held that hypnosis is a state whereby consciousness remains but suggestions reach through consciousness to the subconscious mind. This dual existence, according to Teitelbaum, results in the greater awareness and increased suggestibility of the mind. The greater the depth of the hypnotic state, the more passive consciousness becomes; therefore the subconscious accepts the suggestions more easily. But at all times, contended Teitelbaum, consciousness remains and aids the subconscious in its role.

Perceptual-cognitive Restructuring Theory

Barber (1957a, 1957b, 1958a, 1958b) attributed the effect of hypnotic suggestion to a "perceptual-cognitive restructuring" and contended that the resultant phenomena can be understood in terms of one general principle: "The good subject accepts the hypnotist's words as true statements, he 'perceives' and conceives reality as the operator defines it [1957a, p. 157]." Barber did not believe that the hypnotic subject is in a distinctive and altered state of conscious awareness that is different from his normal self. He believed that successful suggestibility does not depend upon a formal hypnotic induction procedure nor achievement of the so-called hypnotic state, but rather upon the careful selection of people who possess a natural suggestibility, whether in hypnosis or the normal waking state.

Development-interactive Theory

Hilgard (1962) held that basic trust in parent-child relations is the antecedent to hypnotic susceptibility on which conditioning, learning, and role playing build. He combined the psychoanalytic-developmental, the learning and the role-playing theories.

Interactional Theory of Hypnosis

Haley (1958) emphasized the relationship between the hypnotic operator and the subject as they communicate with one another. Haley described the communicative behavior of hypnotic operator and subject in terms of the ways they behave and the ways they qualify that behavior. These two levels of communication function together to define the type of relationship they have, he said. It was Haley's contention that the hypnotic operator communicates two contradictory levels of message to the subject in a situation where the subject must respond, cannot comment on the contradictory requests, and cannot leave the field, thus creating a double bind.

It was Haley's belief that trance behavior takes place when the hypnotic operator controls what sort of relationship he has with the subject and the subject cannot indicate what sort of relationship it is. He considered the perceptual and somatic experiences of the hypnotic subject a product of this kind of relationship with the emphasis on the interaction, which is observable, rather than on the subjective experiences of the subject, which are conjecture.

Three-factor Theory of Hypnosis

Shor (1970) has advanced a three-factor theory to account for hypnosis. His theory postulates that hypnosis is a complex of three separate but complementary psychological processes which are conceived as continuously variable. These three processes are called the dimensions of hypnosis: (1) trance depth, (2) depth of nonconscious involvement, and (3) depth of archaic involvement. Shor defines trance depth as "the extent to which at any given moment in time the true state of affairs is unrepresented in the subject's conscious, phenomenal self-awareness." [p. 91] Depth of nonconscious involvement is defined as "the extent to which at any given moment in time the hypnotic experiences and behaviors are executed by the subject without conscious intention—i.e., without consciously directed motivation, even seemingly in defiance of it." [p. 91] Depth of archaic involvement is defined as "the extent to which at any given moment in time the subject is expressing attitudes, yearnings, and modes of relating to the hypnotist as of a child toward his parents." [p. 92]

CYBERNETIC THEORY OF HYPNOSIS

Skemp (1972) has developed a theory of hypnosis based on the concept of a cybernetic system. The central concept of a cybernetic system is feedback: an activity is controlled, while in progress, by feeding back information about the present state of the system. A cybernetic control system is a goal-seeking system which uses continuous input of information to vary its output adaptively to changing conditions. Successful functioning depends partly on the way in which the information is processed.

According to Skemp, most of the behavior disorders for which people seek help are failures of the patient's control systems. To put these disorders right requires: (1) awareness of the faulty control system, of which the patient is usually unconscious; (2) replacing it with a more effective one; and (3) integrating it with the other control systems.

The cybernetic theory views hypnosis as the progressive takeover of certain of the subject's control systems by the hypnotist, with the aim of obtaining otherwise inaccessible information to enable the patient to do things that he cannot, for some reason, do for himself.

According to the cybernetic theory, the various stages of hypnosis represent progressive stages of the takeover of the subject's control systems. The only point at which the hypnotic operator can enter the feedback loop is as a source of information. The hypnotic operator becomes the main source of information to the subject about the results of his actions, the subject attaching ever-increasing weight to verbal input of information from the hypnotic operator, so that this can eventually override the evidence of his senses (as in hallucinations), other situational data (as in repression), and other approach-avoidance control systems such as pleasure-anxiety.

Each successive stage of hypnotic depth, according to this theory, indicates a new cybernetic system over which the hypnotic operator, replacing the usual sources of information, has gained control. The stage reached is a measure of the subject's suggestibility. A person is suggestible to the extent that he accepts information from outside without subjecting it to the usual processes for testing its consistency with data from other sources. In hypnosis, these other sources are inhibited, so increased suggestibility necessarily results.

Conclusion   Some of these theories can be summarily discarded. For instance, there is no evidence to indicate that suggestibility or the hypnotic state are symptomatic of a pathological condition. Similarly, the theory that hypnosis in humans is identical to states of immobilization as seen in animals is no longer tenable. Also, there is ample evidence to contradict any hypothesis that hypnosis is a form of sleep or a state of unconsciousness. The theory that hypnosis is a state of dissociation was discredited when it was demonstrated that there is a hyperacuity of the senses during hypnosis, and that amnesia can be removed by suggestions of the hypnotic operator and that it does not always occur spontaneously. Finally, the animal magnetism theory was discredited even in Mesmer's time. Although research findings have found these hypotheses to be untenable, there are present-day proponents of each of these discredited theories.

Although the neurophysiological theories may account for the hypnotic state per se, they cannot account for the majority of phenomena associated with hypnosis. When trying to explain hypnosis in terms of hypersuggestibility, there remains the task of explaining how hypersuggestibility comes about, what its nature is, and how it can bring about all of the phenomena associated with hypnosis. The same can be said in relation to the superconcentration of the mind theory and the theory of hypnosis as a bypassing of the critical faculty.

Many of the other theories, such as the conditioned response theory and the ideomotor activity and inhibition theory, account for hypnosis in part, but not for the entire phenomenon. This is also true of the psychoanalytic and psychosomatic theories of hypnosis. None of these theories accounts for all hypnotic phenomena; for instance, the psychoanalytical view of hypnosis as a form of transference does not account for such phenomena as self-hypnosis.

Many of the recent contributions to the theoretical aspect of hypnosis represent a merging of two or more existing theories belonging under one of the other classifications. These tend to emphasize the double nature of hypnosis as a physiological and a psychological phenomenon. The strong point of many of these theories is the fact that they do recognize the physiological and psychological aspects of hypnosis. But, for the most part, they have the same weaknesses as others that have been examined, for in most instances they combine two or more existing theories without eliminating the weaknesses that these already possess.

It seems a fair appraisal to state that each theory of hypnosis, with the exception of those that have been disproven by research findings, has adequately explained some aspects of hypnosis, but none has provided a satisfactory explanation of all its properties. Up to a certain point, each theory accounts quite well for certain known facts, but sooner or later fails in the face of other facts. In some instances, the weakness is due to the fact that the theoretical constructs are so general and abstract as to explain little if anything or not be measurable. Others have centered their theories around a phenomenon that is itself poorly understood and that tends to be too general. Still others have focused on a specific and tangible enough phenomenon, but have limited themselves too much to the overall aspects of hypnosis.

A comprehensive theory of hypnosis must not only take care of the general, but must also account for the particular. It should explain the induced hypnotic state, self-hypnosis, mass hypnosis, waking states of suggestibility, induced positive and negative hallucinations, hypnagogic reveries, posthypnotic phenomena and so forth. In addition, it must account for the temporariness of hypnosis and the spontaneous fluctuations that occur as well as the wide individual differences in hypnotic susceptibility. Whatever truth may be found in any existing theory will have to be taken into consideration by a comprehensive theory. It should go without saying that every aspect of such a theory must satisfy the rigorous criteria of the scientific method.

Chapter 2.

Hypnotic
Phenomena

For purposes of convenience, hypnotic phenomena will be divided into the following categories: induction phenomena; spontaneous phenomena; phenomena associated with alterations in the voluntary muscles; phenomena associated with alterations in the involuntary muscles, organs and glands; phenomena associated with alterations in the sense organs; psychological phenomena associated with memory, mental activity, emotions and ideational processes; and posthypnotic phenomena.

INDUCTION PHENOMENA

A number of psychological changes are present during the induction phase. Immobilization of the body and repetition of the hypnotic operator's suggestions produces a gradual narrowing of sensory avenues.

Feelings of relaxation increase as a person goes deeper into hypnosis. This bodily relaxation is experienced internally by increasing feelings of bodily warmth and feelings of heaviness.

Spontaneous thoughts and feelings during the induction phase are prominent during the first few hypnotic sessions, but after the subject has been conditioned to enter hypnosis rapidly, he will not be as aware of his emotions or thought processes during induction.

With induction techniques utilizing eye fixation, some subjects experience visual illusions or hallucinations. Kaleidoscopic patterns

15

or abstract forms appear to symbolize the monotony and rhythm of the induction process. Feelings of relaxation are often expressed as the sense of floating on a cloud or sinking into a foam rubber mattress. Some subjects report illusions of the room widening or getting smaller.

Sensations of ego dissolution are common during hypnotic induction. Some subjects have reported such feelings as being separated into fragments: they were standing in a corner of the room looking at themselves sitting in the chair. According to Wolberg (1948), these sensations are probably the psychologic components of regression with beginning dissolution of ego boundaries.

It is common for the subject to experience intense emotions during the induction phase. The intensity of the emotions is due in part to the release of inhibitions with liberation of repressed feelings and in part to the subject's own interpretation of the hypnotic experience. The quality of mood may vary from ecstasy or joy to fear or anxiety.

Objective phenomena during the induction phase depend upon the type of induction technique employed. With induction techniques utilizing eye fixation, the following phenomena may be observed: dilation of the pupils, increased lacrimation, the whites of the eyes getting red or pink, blinking and involuntary drooping of the eyelids and immobilization of the head, neck and skeletal system.

Spontaneous Phenomena

Spontaneous phenomena are due to the fact that hypnosis dissolves resistance and makes possible the conscious expression of subconscious impulses. They are also the result of a desire by the subject to comply with the hypnotic operator by manifesting the phenomena which, according to his experience and expectations, he believes will be expected of him.

Common spontaneous phenomena during hypnosis include the recall of memories that had been forgotten in the waking state, sudden awakening, and the development of certain psychosomatic symptoms. For instance, it is a common observation that suggested amnesia may result in spontaneous headaches until the memory that has been forgotten is recalled.

In hysterical subjects, hypnosis may produce spontaneous fits of uncontrollable laughter or crying.

PHENOMENA ASSOCIATED WITH ALTERATIONS IN VOLUNTARY MUSCLES

During hypnosis, the movements of the voluntary muscles can either be inhibited or excited.

Relaxation Suggestions of muscular relaxation induce a pronounced disinclination to move the limbs; as the hypnotic state deepens, muscular tonus diminishes.

Paralysis of muscle groups There is actually no loss of motor power; rather there is a temporary suspension of tonicity and motion. Hypnotic paralysis may involve small muscle groups, such as the eyelids, or larger groups, such as the limbs or trunk. The paralysis may be of a flaccid or spastic nature; it is based entirely on the subject's conception of how a paralyzed person behaves.

Catalepsy Catalepsy refers to a condition of muscular rigidity in which the limbs or body remain passively in any position in which they are placed.

Automatic movements Automatic movements are movements of any group of muscles without conscious control. Two of the most frequently utilized automatic movements are arm levitation and rotation of the hands around each other. The hypnotic subject would be trained to produce automatic movements prior to the utilization of automatic writing or automatic drawing.

Increased muscular performance In hypnosis, the subject can perform tasks with much less discomfort and fatigue than in the normal waking state. We all have considerable reserves of power that can be tapped in hypnosis. It is important to realize, however, that no one can be made to exceed his own individual capacity.

PHENOMENA ASSOCIATED WITH ALTERATIONS IN INVOLUNTARY MUSCLES, ORGANS AND GLANDS

Many bodily functions are outside voluntary control and are regulated by the subconscious mind acting through the thalamus on the autonomic nervous system. The circulatory, respiratory, alimentary and excretory systems and the endocrine glands are for the most part regulated in this manner. The subconscious mind has the power to inhibit or excite the autonomic nervous system. Since the subconscious mind becomes more accessible to suggestion in hypnosis, much of the influence exerted under hypnosis becomes explicable.

The heart   The heart rate can be accelerated or retarded by suggestion in hypnosis.

The blood-vessels   Hypnotic suggestion can exercise a certain amount of influence on the blood-vessels. Many investigators have reported that the smaller arteries and capillaries are almost invariably contracted in deep hypnosis so that even deep wounds tend to produce little or no hemorrhage. Experimental studies have also been reported in which increases and decreases in body temperature have been achieved by hypnotic suggestion. The blood pressure can also be influenced by hypnotic suggestion. Suggestions of relaxation and calmness will lower the blood pressure and pulse rate, whereas suggestions of excitement will raise them.

The respiratory system   Shallow, diaphragmatic breathing usually is associated with lighter stages of hypnosis, while slow, deep abdominal breathing is characteristic of deeper stages. Hypnotic suggestion can produce considerable variations of both respiration rate and respiratory excursion. Hartland (1966) reported that increases in pulmonary ventilation up to fifty percent have been obtained in a resting hypnotized subject to whom it had been suggested that heavy work was being performed.

The alimentary system   It has been reported that increased and decreased gastric acidity can be produced by suggestions of enjoyment or disgust. Peristalsis can frequently be influenced by suggestions, and because of this the bowel actions can often be regulated by hypnotic suggestion.

The secretions   Secretion of saliva and perspiration have been induced by hypnotic suggestion. The eyes can be caused to water if it is suggested to the hypnotized subject that he is smelling an onion. Also, lactation can be facilitated and the secretion of milk greatly increased by hypnotic suggestion.

Changes in metabolism   The blood-sugar level can be increased or decreased by means of hypnotic suggestion. A fall in blood-sugar results when a deeply hypnotized subject is told that he hasn't eaten anything for several days. If he is then told that he is eating an imaginary meal of rich pastry, a rise in blood-sugar will occur.

Anatomical and biochemical changes   There are a number of organic changes that can be brought about by means of hypnosis. Menstruation can often be induced or stopped by hypnotic suggestion. Blisters have been produced by suggesting to a deeply hypnotized subject that a pencil being pressed upon his skin was a red-hot poker and that it was burning his skin. There have been numerous reports of the modification of allergic reactions by means of direct hypnotic suggestion.

PHENOMENA ASSOCIATED WITH ALTERATIONS IN THE SENSE ORGANS

Sensory hyperesthesia   Sensory hyperesthesia refers to increased acuity of the senses. On suggestion, a hypnotic subject may be made to distinguish variations in texture and temperature that could not be differentiated in the normal waking state.

Hypnoanalgesia   Hypnoanalgesia is the hypnotically produced absence of sensibility to pain. It is characterized by a lack of startle reaction and facial grimaces.

Hypnoanesthesia   Hypnoanesthesia refers to the hypnotically produced absence of feeling. It may be total or partial.

Paresthesia   Paresthesia refers to abnormal, distorted, or wrongly localized sensation. Among the paresthesias that are relatively easy to suggest are numbness, tingling, itching, burning, sensations of coldness, and increased sensitivity to stimuli of pain, pressure and temperature. Paresthesias of the special senses include those of vision, known as photomata, in the form of flashes of light and color; of distorted taste sensations, paraguesia, whereby the hypnotized subject's sense of taste can be so modified that a glass of water may taste like wine; and of distorted sensations of smell, parosmia. A hypnotized subject's sense of smell can be modified so that if a bottle of ammonia is held under his nose with the suggestion that it is perfume, he will be convinced that it is perfume.

Positive hallucinations   A positive hallucination is a sense experience in the absence of appropriate sensory stimuli. Hallucinations can be produced in connection with any of the five senses. A good hypnotic subject can be induced to see a person, to hear music or to smell perfume in the absence of any external stimuli.

Negative hallucinations   A negative hallucination is the absence of a sense experience in the presence of appropriate sensory stimuli. Negative hallucinations are possible only in the deepest state of somnambulism. When successful, the hypnotic subject is unable to recognize the presence of either an object or a person with which he is confronted.

Psychological Phenomena

The psychological phenomena characteristic of the hypnotic state will be discussed under the following headings: memory, mental activity, the emotions and ideational processes.

Memory   All memories are stored in the brain and most of them can be recovered when the proper association pathways are stimulated. The following hypnotic phenomena are related to memory: hypermnesia, age regression and revivification.

Hypermnesia refers to an increase in memory recall greater than that achieved at nonhypnotic levels. A good hypnotic subject can recall memories that have been entirely forgotten for many years.

In age regression, the subject is brought back to some earlier period of his life. He can remember all of the incidents of his life of that particular period and can describe them vividly and accurately. Although the subject goes back into the past and may describe past events with considerable feeling, he does so with an adult intelligence and personality and uses the past tense in relating the recalled events.

Revivification is a type of regression in which the client returns to a former point in time and actually relives his past experiences. He speaks and behaves as a child and experiences the emotions evoked by the event in the way that a child of that age experiences emotion. In revivification, all memories following the age to which the subject has regressed are forgotten.

Mental Activity   The following phenomena will be discussed: rapport, the sense and judgment of time and personality changes.

Rapport refers to the state of affinity existing between subject and hypnotic operator and is present at the very onset of hypnosis. It tends to prevent the hypnotic subject from responding to any stimuli other than those arising from the hypnotic operator unless he instructs the subject otherwise. Rapport can either be transferred to or shared with another person, should the hypnotic operator so desire.

The human brain has a remarkable capacity to appreciate, condense or expand time. Everyone has an "alarm clock" in his brain that is capable of judging time with extraordinary accuracy. In hypnosis, the subject is able to judge the passage of time more accurately than in the normal waking state because the subconscious processes regulating the time sense can be controlled by hypnotic suggestion. If the hypnotized subject is asked to perform a task after a specified number of minutes, he will usually do it with a fairly high degree of accuracy. Also, the hypnotic subject will perform an act as the result of a posthypnotic suggestion, after a specified time interval.

The condensation or expansion of time by means of hypnotic suggestion is known as time distortion. Time distortion can be induced readily in somnambulistic subjects. One minute of subjective time can be equated with ten minutes of clock or chronologic time (time expansion), or ten minutes of clock time can be condensed to one minute of subjective time (time condensation). Cooper and Erickson (1954) gave a complete description of this most interesting and therapeutically valuable hypnotic phenomenon.

A somnambulistic subject can be convinced by means of hypnotic suggestion that he is a totally different personality. If several different personalities are suggested, each successive personality change is usually accompanied by a loss of memory of that which preceded it.

The Emotions   The general feelings of a subject can be readily influenced by hypnotic suggestion. Emotions such as joy, sadness, love, hate, fear and anger can readily be induced in somnambulistic subjects and may alternate very quickly. Any mood can be artificially induced in hypnosis if a specific situation is suggested which tends to arouse that mood.

Ideational Processes   Among hypnotic techniques utilized during hypnoanalysis are free association, dream induction, automatic writing, drawing and the induction of experimental conflicts. All of these hypnotic procedures involve complicated ideational processes.

Spontaneous fantasy and imagery may be increased in hypnotic subjects. The content of the fantasies will depend upon the meaning of hypnosis to the subject and upon his aptitude for symbolizing his experiences.

Upon suggestion, the associative and symbolic functions can be eliminated or distorted, with these resulting disorders of association and symbolic functions:

Dissociation: the ability of a hypnotic subject to detach himself from his immediate environment.

Aphasia: impairment or loss of the ability to communicate and understand language symbols.

Agraphia: partial or complete inability to understand or express ideas in writing.

Alexia: inability to read correctly.

Upon suggestion these disturbances of attention can be induced:

Aprosexia: the inability to concentrate on specified activities in the environment.

Hyperprosexia: a morbid focusing of attention on a restricted area.

POSTHYPNOTIC PHENOMENA

The following posthypnotic phenomena will be discussed: spontaneous phenomena, posthypnotic amnesia, and posthypnotic suggestions.

Spontaneous Phenomena Immediately upon coming out of the hypnotic state, the subject undergoes an ego synthesis, with restoration of ego boundaries, a reorientation in time and place, and reestablishment of volitional control.

Posthypnotic Amnesia Subjects suffer from a loss of memory in the waking state as the result of the suggestion to forget, given while the subject was in the hypnotic state.

Posthypnotic Suggestions Any phenomenon induced during hypnosis may also be executed posthypnotically upon suggestion. In most cases, posthypnotic suggestions are effective only after the subject has developed a deep state of hypnosis which has been followed by amnesia. Posthypnotic suggestion is invaluable in the therapeutic application of hypnosis. It is also useful in facilitating the future induction of hypnosis by means of posthypnotic conditioning for immediate reinduction upon cue.

Part Two
Induction of
Hypnosis

Chapter 3.

Favorable Conditions for Hypnotic Induction

The client must have confidence and trust in the hypnotic operator. If the subject is apprehensive and doesn't have complete trust in the operator, he won't allow himself to go beyond a certain point, most probably not beyond a very light stage of hypnosis. Everyhing that is done or said from the moment the subject enters the hypnotic operator's office is of importance in instilling confidence and trust. Since the effectiveness of the hypnotic induction depends to a large degree upon the strength of the interpersonal relationship, sufficient time must be spent in building up this trust and in getting to know the subject.

A comfortable position is necessary in order for the subject to go into hypnosis. The subject should be allowed to assume whatever position is comfortable for him. He should be told that if at any time during hypnosis he begins to feel uncomfortable, he will be able to change his position without interfering with his level of relaxation. It is good to advise the subject to loosen any clothing that is too tight, such as a tie or belt, as this will prevent him from attaining maximum relaxation. Also, the subject should be advised to go to the restroom if he feels the need before the session begins as pressure on the bladder acts as a detriment to relaxation.

The room temperature in the hypnotic consulting room should be comfortable, neither too warm nor too cool. If the client is sitting in a draft, it will interfere with the hypnotic induction. The ideal temperature will vary from client to client; it is a good practice to ask the client whether or not the room temperature is comfortable for him.

All distractions should be eliminated and all outside noises should be discouraged. The hypnotic operator should be very observant and try to discover anything that may interfere with the hypnotic induction. Noises within the room, such as the ticking of a clock, will be disturbing for certain clients. If the distraction or noise is beyond control, such as the noise from passing cars or the noise from a typewriter in an outer office, the hypnotic operator can make effective use of these noises by telling the client that with every sound of a car or with every click of a typewriter, he will become more and more relaxed.

Background music is often helpful as an aid to hypnotic induction. Care should be taken to ascertain the client's preference in musical selections and to determine whether the background music is an aid or a hindrance to induction for that particular client. If music is used, it should be soft and soothing instrumental music with even tempo and pitch and should be played as a musical background for hypnotic induction.

Stirring the client's imagination is helpful.

Chapter 4.

Necessary Considerations in Hypnotic Induction

The following considerations are necessary for the successful induction of hypnosis: the education of the client, the client's expectations, the qualifications of the client, the conditioning of the client, and the qualifications of the hypnotic operator.

THE EDUCATION OF THE CLIENT

Suggestions and techniques must be tailored to the client. A superstitious, uneducated person will respond quite differently from the way a sophisticated scientist will respond. The words used in a suggestion must conform to the client's familiarity with the language. The more limited the education of the client, the more careful the hypnotic operator will have to be in his choice of words.

The hypnotic operator will have to use different approaches with children and adults. The induction procedure can be in the form of a game with a child. Chapter Seven includes a number of induction techniques for use with children.

Dr. Bernard Gindes, in *New Concepts of Hypnosis* (1953), gives a good example of the importance of considering the educational background of the subject. He cites a case where a colleague was working with a difficult subject and kept repeating the suggestion that the subject's body was becoming more and more lethargic. After more than an hour of futile effort, the subject opened his eyes and asked, "What is lethargic, anyway?"

27

The Expectations of the Client

What the subject expects to happen in hypnosis is of utmost importance. Each person reacts in the way he expects to react. Many persons expect to fall asleep and become unconscious. When this doesn't happen, they will often deny that they were in hypnosis, even if they were in a deep state of hypnosis. Once the subject has experienced what it is like to be hypnotized, his belief is strengthened and he knows what to expect. If fear and doubt were retarding factors before, they will have become extinguished through the pleasant experience of the complete physical and mental relaxation of the hypnotic state.

Qualifications of the Client

The following qualifications of the client are extremely important considerations in hypnotic induction: belief, expectation, imagination, concentration, freedom from doubt and fear, and motivation.

In order for the induction procedure to be successful, the subject must have complete belief in hypnosis as a genuine phenomenon; he must believe in his ability to be hypnotized; and he must believe in the integrity and ability of the hypnotic operator.

As mentioned previously, the subject's preconceived expectations concerning hypnosis are very important and should be taken into consideration by the hypnotic operator before attempting induction.

It is essential that the client be able to use his imagination in order for suggestions to be effective. In hypnosis, mental images are modified as products of the imagination. Mental images can be modified to such an extent that an event from the client's past can be summoned, and, in accordance with the remembrance, the client is able to relive the recreated experience with the same emotional feeling that he experienced when the event first took place. A hypnotized person will enact a suggestion only if it has been enforced previously, either in reality or in imagination.

The client must be able to concentrate on the suggestions given to him by the hypnotic operator and to wrap his mind around the idea that is presented; he must accept it wholeheartedly in order for him to enter the hypnotic state. The hypnotic state is characterized by heightened concentration; the deeper the person goes into hypnosis, the greater the concentration.

The client must be free from doubt and fear in order to go into hypnosis. He must believe wholeheartedly that the suggestion is going to be effective, in order for it to be so. He must accept the suggestion given to him by the hypnotic operator and in turn give it to himself, believing completely that it will be effective. If there is the slightest doubt or fear on the part of the client, the suggestion will not be effective, and he will not enter hypnosis.

The client has to want to go into hypnosis. The hypnotic operator should discover what the client's motives are for wanting to go into hypnosis. If the motives are not good ones, then hypnosis should not be chosen for treatment. The better the motives and the stronger the motivation on the part of the client, the better the chances for a successful hypnotic induction.

THE CONDITIONING OF THE CLIENT

The client must be conditioned toward high expectations. When one suggestion is effective, the client's expectation is stronger that the next suggestion will take effect. That is why it is so important that the hypnotic operator compound suggestions. Any technique, in order to be truly effective, must include the pyramiding of expectations. Many individuals respond to hypnotic suggestions in direct proportion to the number of suggestions given to them. Suggestion One becomes stronger when Suggestion Two is given; Suggestion One and Two become stronger when Suggestion Three is given, and so on.

The hypnotic operator is a salesman in a very real sense. He must sell his product to the client. The only way to sell hypnosis to the client is to convince him that he can be hypnotized, and the only way to do that is by inducing the hypnotic state in him. The hypnotic operator must be thoroughly convinced of the value of his product if he expects to sell his client on its value.

Before beginning induction, the hypnotic operator should discuss the common misconceptions of hypnosis and give the client a clear, concise definition of hypnosis. He should give the client examples of hypnosis in everyday life and a comparison of hypnosis with the twilight state a person is in just before waking up in the morning and just before falling asleep at night. The hypnotic operator should also assure the client that nothing dangerous nor embarrassing will be done to him.

Qualifications of the Hypnotic Operator

There are a number of qualifications for the successful hypnotic operator. The following are essential for true proficiency: self-assurance and confidence, keen observation, an ability to utilize imagination and belief to the utmost, an ability to convey the impression of authority and prestige, a comforting and dynamic voice, thorough training and experience, and an ability to present suggestions plausibly and logically.

The first aim of the beginner in professional hypnosis should be self-assurance and confidence, as this is the most important qualification of the successful hypnotic operator. The hypnotic operator must be able to enlist the confidence and cooperation of the client. He must avoid hesitancy in his presentation, and he must be prepared for the unexpected and know what he is doing every step of the way. The client will correlate hesitancy, confusion or surprise with lack of ability.

The successful hypnotic operator has developed a keen sense of observation. Each client will present different personality traits, attitudes, experiences and needs. Awareness of all of these individual differences and knowing how to deal with them and use them to advantage is essential for success.

The good hypnotic operator has the ability to utilize imagination and belief to the utmost. He is really a dream pilot, in the sense that he is able to effectively stimulate and guide the client's imagination. In order to do this successfully, the hypnotic operator must have a well-developed imagination himself.

The hypnotic operator must be able to give the impression of authority and prestige. This doesn't mean that he should be authoritarian or abrupt. It does mean that he should give the impression that he knows what he is doing, that he is in complete control of the situation and that he conducts himself in a professional manner. His office should be comfortable and conducive to relaxation. Also, the hypnotic operator should display his diplomas and certificates in open view so that the client can see at a glance that he is qualified. If one has a reputation as a competent hypnotic operator, his clients will be more amenable to his suggestions.

A comforting and dynamic voice is essential for success. It is a good practice for a therapist to record his inductions in the early stages of his hypnotic training and to play it back when he is alone. He will be able to learn a great deal from this: if his voice is too loud or too raspy, then he will have to work at cultivating a more smooth, soothing voice. By listening to tape recordings of his inductions, he will also discover whether he sounds anxious or hesitant in his delivery. Hypnosis is an art as well as a science. Knowledge of hypnotic techniques is not enough. A successful hypnotic operator is one who has mastered hypnotic techniques and procedures and voice intonations by means of constant study and practice.

Thorough training and experience is necessary in order to be a truly competent hypnotic operator. The competent hypnotic operator will have a mastery of a number of methods and techniques; he will have read widely in the hypnosis literature and be conversant on all important aspects of the field; he will have had a considerable amount of practical experience; he will learn from his failures and constantly seek to improve his techniques and will keep abreast of current developments in the field by means of continuing education.

The successful hypnotic operator has the ability to present suggestions plausibly and logically. Also, he is able to explain how suggestion works and how the various phenomena develop, in order to gain the client's understanding and acceptance.

In order to be truly proficient, the hypnotic operator must have a good understanding of the meaning of words, and he must be able to adjust his vocabulary to the chronological and educational level of the client.

One of the most important qualifications of the successful hypnotic operator is great patience. Many conditions require a great deal of patience before success can follow. The hypnotic operator must remain even tempered, calm, and well composed in the face of resistance, the unexpected and failure.

Chapter 5.

Hindrances to Hypnotic Induction

The attitude of the subject may be a hindrance to hypnotic induction. A critical, skeptical or analytic attitude is not conducive to successful hypnosis. Hypnosis is a consent state: it requires complete cooperation on the part of the subject. Since hypnosis is a state of mind in which the critical faculty is bypassed and selective thinking is established, skepticism or analytical thinking will prevent an individual from entering the hypnotic state.

Hypnosis is contraindicated for the following types of individuals: prepsychotic, latent homosexual, the pseudointellectual, individuals of low intelligence, individuals with a serious lack of integration of the personality, and all of those who are perversely motivated toward hypnosis.

The motivation of the patient who comes specifically seeking treatment by hypnosis requires close scrutiny by the hypnotic operator. The following are the most common unconscious motivations that lead people to seek hypnosis:

Magic. A number of patients consult a hypnotherapist for the express purpose of seeking hypnosis for the relief of their symptoms. They may have read about hypnosis in a newspaper or magazine article and decided that hypnosis must be the treatment they require. This type of patient sees in hypnosis the means of magic. He expects removal of his symptoms by means of hypnotic suggestion without assuming any responsibility on his part or working through to the underlying causes of the symptoms.

33

Ideas of influence. Paranoid schizophrenics frequently seek hypnosis and often rationalize their ideas of influence into the belief that they have been hypnotized. The prepsychotic schizophrenic who seeks hypnosis is much more difficult to assess. Such patients may deny any ideas of influence but often make persistent demands to be hypnotized. They experience vague ideas of influence which aren't conceived clearly in the patient's conscious awareness. It is extremely important that these patients be recognized! Hypnosis with them may precipitate an active psychotic process and may also lead to the hypnotherapist's being actively involved in the patient's delusions.

Rationalization for keeping symptoms. The chronic neurotic who is deriving a great deal of secondary gain from his symptoms and who has no intention of changing his state may come seeking treatment and say, "I have such and such a symptom and I have come to see if you can hypnotize me." This type of patient is convinced that he will not be able to be hypnotized. His motivation amounts to a rationalization for keeping his symptoms. Hypnotic treatment with such a patient is sure to fail as long as he is convinced that he cannot be hypnotized.

Masculine-aggressive women. Patients with latent aggression come for hypnosis with a similar "hypnotize-me-if-you-can" attitude. Their general motivation for hypnosis is to demonstrate that they can't be overpowered by a man. Attempts at hypnotic induction will usually fail with this type of patient because hypnosis is a consent state. If the individual is in any way defensive, then hypnosis will fail.

The last hope motivation patient. This type of person usually has had a great deal of illness and a great number of operations, all without relief. He has lost faith in medicine and psychotherapy. Hypnosis is the last resort in the fight against chronic illness. This type of motivation makes hypnosis extremely difficult. Although this type of person comes for treatment, he comes without hope. His expectance is zero. Before the hypnotic state can be successfully induced, both hope and expectancy must be rekindled. These unconscious motivations for hypnotic treatment do not usually occur in pure form. More often, they form a background upon which conscious reasons operate.

We have discussed some of the unconscious motivations for hypnotic treatment. The patient may also have unconscious motivations against hypnosis, which fall into one of three groups: (1) The insecure—frightened of being overpowered. These individuals lack the necessary trust to surrender themselves. (2) Aggression—if the aggressive person regards hypnosis as authoritative, he will avoid it because it will mobilize his aggression. Also, his aggression doesn't allow him to accept passive hypnosis. (3) Hypnosis as sexuality—this is characterized by a mental attitude according to which any close or intimate relationship is regarded as erotic.

Various unconscious motivations may come into operation to prevent the onset of hypnosis. Meares (1954) described various unconscious defenses that come into operation to prevent the onset of hypnosis. Clinically, it is important to recognize defenses as they manifest themselves so that appropriate countermeasures may be taken. The following are the unconscious defenses against hypnosis as described by Meares:

Restlessness. Most often seen when a progressive relaxation induction is used. It may manifest itself in fidgeting, coughing, shivering, etc. If the defense is poorly developed, it should be met directly by continuing suggestions of relaxation. However, if the restlessness is persistent, an immediate change should be made to another technique. The patient's defenses should be turned against him, i.e., when hand fidgeting is a prominent feature, induction by arm levitation is often satisfactory.

Negativism. The patient defends himself against hypnosis by doing the opposite of what is suggested. The important thing is that the patient is influenced by suggestion, although in the wrong direction. The defense must be circumvented in order for hypnotic induction to be successful. This can usually be done by inducing repetitive movements.

Simulation. The patient tries to avoid hypnosis by consciously carrying out all suggestions. This type of defense is recognized by the promptness with which suggestions are followed. An immediate response to a suggestion should make the operator think of simulation. When this defense is recognized, it is a mistake to point it out to the subject and to start again. The subject should be allowed to maintain his simulation. Suggestions are continued and the patient is led to believe that the hypnotic operator thinks him properly hypnotized. This is continued for several sessions until it is observed that movements have become slower and lose some of the natural ease of voluntary movement. Gradually challenges are introduced. When it is gauged from the response to suggestions that the patient is really hypnotized, he is strongly challenged.

Sleep. This defense is most common when induction is made by arm levitation. The hypnotic operator should convert to hypnosleep (hypnosis attached to sleep) and give the patient a posthypnotic suggestion to awaken within a specified time and then convert back to the sleep state.

Symptoms as a defense. For example, a patient with asthma develops a severe attack just at the critical stage of induction.

Defense by depreciation. An attempt is made to allay anxiety by depreciating the situation, i.e., patient grins or giggles, shakes his head, etc. The hypnotic operator should remain calm and continue suggestions.

Startle reaction. The patient awakens with a terrific start. Sometimes it occurs only once. The hypnotic operator should change to an active technique.

Turning away. When hypnosis is being induced by eye fixation, the patient sometimes defends himself by suddenly turning away or refusing to look. When this defense is encountered, the hypnotic operator should change to arm levitation, which usually succeeds.

The successful use of hypnosis is dependent upon the ability of the hypnotic operator to recognize the various defenses and to take appropriate counteraction. The motivation for the defenses is the patient's anxiety at the threat of loss of ego control. The motivation for these defenses is very much reduced by careful attention to rapport, passivity and surrender before attempting hypnotic induction.

Pipe or cigarette smoking by the hypnotic operator may be objectionable. Subjects with severe coughs or head colds should not be induced for the first time, as they are often bothered by coughing or sneezing.

The posture of the subject is important. The back of the head should be well supported, as neck strain interferes with induction. The best type of chair to use is a reclining vibrating chair. Tight clothing should be loosened prior to the hypnotic induction. Anything that distracts the subject or makes him uncomfortable will interefere with the hypnotic induction.

Chapter 6.

Methods of
Hypnotic Induction

All of the methods of hypnotic induction that I use and teach my students in hypnotherapy classes are verbal induction techniques, with the exception of induction by repetitive movement, which is a combination of verbal induction and physical contact. The entire procedure in verbal induction is conducted through the medium of spoken instructions and reinforcements delivered by the hypnotic operator.

In discussing the advantages of verbal induction, London (1967) stated:

> Complete reliance on verbal communication for the induction of hypnosis has the advantages of freeing the hypnotist from much concern with paraphernalia, permitting maximum flexibility of communication from hypnotist to subject, both in terms of variety and detail of hypnotic instructions, and presenting a more direct introduction to what the hypnotic situation will ordinarily be like than do other methods.

Verbal induction techniques are the most commonly used and physical contact methods are generally ancillary to them. London (1967) very cogently and clearly showed why verbal induction techniques are the most widely used of all the modes of induction in his discussion of the flexibility and importance of verbal induction techniques:

> The great flexibility inherent in verbal inductions permits words to serve as facilitators and substitutes for physical and sensory manipulations . . . perhaps most important to the use of hypnosis for

psychological purposes is the power that verbal induction alone has to channel the multiple response capacities of the subject into any of the many behaviors that are of interest either therapeutically or scientifically. Though some physiological changes may be inevitable in the achievement of a hypnotic state, it is only through verbal induction techniques that precise changes can be produced. Age regression, trance logic, hypermnesia, and posthypnotic amnesia may all occasionally occur spontaneously, but it is only through the medium of verbal instructions that they can be dependably produced . . . it is the most general case that hypnosis involves cognitive changes of behavior, which in turn affect other aspects of behavior. As long as this is true, it goes without saying that verbal processes are the most important ones in the ordinary course of hypnotic induction and of the hypnotic state itself. [1967, pp. 66-67]

PROGRESSIVE RELAXATION INDUCTION

This method of induction depends upon the induction of passivity of mind. It is preferable to have the subject lying upon a couch with his head supported by a pillow.

1. Ask the subject to take three deep breaths, holding each breath for the count of four, opening the eyes wide when inhaling, closing them when exhaling.
2. Give the suggestion of eyelid heaviness each time the eyelids open.
3. Ask the subject to let his eyelids remain closed after exhaling for the third time.
4. Ask the subject to picture himself lying on the beach . . . sunbathing.
5. Give the suggestion that he can feel the soft, warm sand . . . that he can see the blue sky . . . and that he can feel the warmth of the sun on his body.
6. Tell the subject that as he pictures himself lying on the beach, he is to let all the muscles of his body go limp.
7. Ask him to let the muscles of his feet and ankles relax . . . to let them go limp.
8. Then ask him to let the muscles of his calves relax . . . to let them go limp.
9. Then ask him to let his thigh muscles go limp.
10. Suggest a feeling of heaviness in the subject's legs . . . that his legs are beginning to feel as heavy as lead.
11. Tell the subject that as he lets his legs relax completely, he is feeling more and more at peace . . . that his mind is becoming more and more calm and contented.
12. Give the suggestion that he is enjoying this very pleasant, relaxed feeling.

13. Then suggest that the feeling of relaxation is spreading upwards over his whole body.

14. Ask the subject to let his stomach muscles relax . . . to let them go limp.

15. Then ask him to let go of any tightness in his chest . . . his upper back . . . and his lower back . . . to let all of the muscles in his chest and back go limp . . . allowing them to relax completely.

16. Then give the suggestion that he can feel a feeling of heaviness in his body . . . as if his body wants to sink down . . . deeper and deeper into the soft, warm sand.

17. Tell the subject that as he feels his body sinking comfortably into the sand . . . his entire body is becoming more and more relaxed.

18. Suggest that he can feel the heat of the sun on his body.

19. Then give the suggestion that he is feeling warm and comfortable . . . completely at peace . . . and that a pleasant feeling of relaxation is spreading into his neck . . . his shoulders . . . and his arms.

20. Ask the subject to let his neck muscles relax . . . to let them go limp.

21. Then ask him to allow the muscles of his shoulders to relax . . . to let them go limp.

22. Then ask the subject to allow the muscles of his arms to relax . . . to let them go limp . . . and to feel a feeling of heaviness in his arms . . . as if his arms are becoming as heavy as lead.

23. Then ask him to let all of his facial muscles relax completely . . . to let go of any tightness in the corners of his mouth . . . to let his lips part slightly . . . and to let his chin sag and feel pleasantly heavy and relaxed.

24. Then tell the subject that as all of the muscles of his body relax, his breathing continues regularly and deeply . . . deeply within himself.

25. Then tell the subject that in a moment you are going to lift his right arm . . . tell him to let the arm be as heavy and as limp as the rest of his body . . . to let you do all of the work.

26. Then lift his right arm by the wrist with your thumb and middle finger.

27. Suggest that as you release his arm, it will drop limply . . . and that as soon as it touches any part of his body, he will be at least three times more relaxed.

28. Release the arm to see if it falls without assistance.

29. If there is no muscle tonus and if the arm is limp and heavy, proceed with suggestions for deepening by graded responses (see the chapter on training).

30. If the client controls the arm, switch to induction by arm levitation.

INDUCTION BY ARM LEVITATION

All levitation techniques make use of the subject's ideomotor and ideosensory activities. The technique to be presented was developed by Kroger (1963). It has the following advantages over other levitation techniques: the subject is motivated each step of the way; the subject is not rushed, and he is convinced that the responses result from the operator's suggestions.

The following are the steps for the induction by arm levitation:

1. Ask the subject to place his hands on his thighs and to look down at his hands as they rest lightly on his thighs.
2. Then ask the subject to press down as hard as he can, as if he were pushing his legs and feet through the floor.
3. Suggest that he press harder and harder.
4. As he presses harder and harder, ask the subject to become aware that he is building up a great amount of tension in his fingers.
5. Give the suggestion that he keep pressing harder and harder.
6. Give the suggestion that he can feel an increased sensitivity in his fingertips.
7. Ask the subject to notice the texture of the cloth of the garment his fingers are touching.
8. Give the suggestion that as he continues to press, he will notice the warmth of his body as it comes through his clothing.
9. Tell the subject that the opposite of the tension he is building up in his fingers is relaxation.
10. Tell the subject that any time he wishes to relax, all he has to do is close his eyes and visualize that one of the fingers on either the right hand or the left hand is getting lighter than all the others.
11. Tell the subject that if he really wants to relax, one of the fingers on either the left hand or the right hand is actually getting lighter than all the others.
12. Tell the subject that one of the fingers will begin to move on either the left or the right hand.
13. As you notice movement in a finger say: "I notice that the (name the finger) of the right (or left) hand is beginning to lift. It's lifting . . . lifting . . . lifting."
14. Give the suggestion that as that finger gets lighter than all of the other fingers, the other fingers of that hand can begin to lift.
15. Give the suggestion that very soon the subject is going to notice a floating, soothing sensation.

16. Remark that the right (or left) hand is lifting in the direction of his face—lifting . . . lifting . . . lifting.
17. Ask the subject to give himself the following suggestion: "With each motion that my arm lifts upward, I will go deeper and deeper relaxed; my arm is lifting, not because it has to, but because it wants to. I will soon reach a deep state, a deep state of relaxation."
18. Ask the subject to visualize a balloon tied around his wrist.
19. Then ask him to visualize three balloons tugging at his wrist.
20. Then suggest that the arm is lifting as the balloons rise into the air.
21. Give the subject the suggestion that the moment any portion of his hand touches any portion of his face, that will be a signal for him to drop into an even deeper state of hypnosis, and that his arm will drop limply into his lap.
22. Give the suggestion that as his arm lifts more and more, he is going deeper and deeper into hypnosis.
23. Tell the subject that if he learns these simple suggestions, then he can learn the other suggestions that are so necessary for complete physical and mental relaxation.
24. Tell the subject that as the hand draws closer and closer to his face, he is to think of that wonderful feeling of relaxation that is going to come over his body as soon as any part of his hand touches any part of his face.
25. As soon as the subject's hand touches his face and his arm drops limply into his lap, give the suggestion that he is much more deeply relaxed.
26. Tell the subject that you are going to lift his arm and that if he really wishes to go deeper, he will just let it drop into his lap with a thud when you let go of it.
27. Tell the subject that you will let go on the count of three.
28. Count slowly. One . . . two . . . three . . . thud!
29. Tell the subject that as long as his hands and arms remain in that position, he will continue to go deeper and deeper into relaxation.

INDUCTION BY REPETITIVE MOVEMENT

This method is used with those clients who show negativistic behavior. When one thing is suggested, they tend to do the opposite. Negativistic behavior of this nature is a defense, but is usually below the level of conscious awareness.

The following steps should be followed for induction of hypnosis by repetitive movement:

1. Take the subject's arm by the wrist with the thumb and middle

finger, and place his elbow on the arm of the chair with his arm upwards and fingers pointing toward the ceiling.

2. Move the subject's arm slowly . . . backwards and forwards.
3. As you slowly move the subject's arm backwards and forwards, ask him to imagine a piece of cord tied around his wrist . . . and that someone at each end of the cord is pulling his arm . . . first backwards . . . then forwards.
4. Ask the subject to continue to picture that piece of cord tied round his wirst . . . pulling his arm slowly . . . backwards . . . and forwards, and that as he does so he will find that when you release his wrist, it will feel as if that piece of cord is still tied to his wrist . . . still pulling his arm . . . backwards . . . and forwards.
5. Tell the subject that his arm will go on moving . . . entirely on its own . . . backwards and forwards . . . until you tell it to stop.
6. Tell the subject that he won't try to make it move and he won't try to stop it from moving, but will just let it go on moving on . . . until you tell it to stop.
7. When the arm is moving freely, tell the subject that his level of hypnosis is becoming deeper, timing this so that you repeat the word *deeper* on each alternate forward movement of his arm.
8. After six automatic movements forwards and backwards, tell the subject to stop and put his arm back on the arm of the chair.
9. Then tell the subject that as his arm touches the arm of the chair, he is falling into an even deeper state of hypnosis.

THE DYNAMIC METHOD OF INDUCTION

This method of hypnotic induction was developed by Meares (1960). It involves an outlook on the induction of hypnosis that is quite different from the classical approaches. The theoretical basis for this method is that suggestibility is a dynamic function of the psyche, in contrast to the classic concept of suggestibility as a fixed and rigid facet of the personality. The classic approach is static, in that it makes no allowance for the psychodynamic mechanisms that may be working to prevent the onset of hypnosis. Meares (1960) stated:

The dynamic method is based on two hypotheses: that hypnosis involves a primitive state of mental functioning and that the patient who consciously desires hypnosis is prevented from returning to this primitive state of mental functioning by the activity of unconscious psychological defense mechanisms. The dynamic method aims to allow hypnosis by the circumvention of these defenses. [p. 206]

According to Meares, the exact form of the initial suggestions is unimportant, and as the induction proceeds, the suggestions are determined by the patient's behavior. It is never known at the outset whether or not it will be necessary to use the dynamic method.

The initial induction technique and the accompanying suggestions should be determined by the nature of the patient's defense. If the patient appears to be relaxed, it is best to start with suggestions of relaxation; if he is tense, then it is best to start with arm levitation; if he shows signs of negativism, then it is best to begin with repetitive movement, and so on. If the subject accepts the initial suggestions, then the operator can proceed with the particular technique being used and there is no need to employ the dynamic method. However, if the subject shows sustained defenses, then the operator should switch.

An example will clarify the procedure. Let us suppose that the operator begins with the progressive relaxation induction technique. If the operator observes that the subject is restless, he should direct the subject's attention to his restlessness with a view to using it in the hypnotic induction. If the operator notices a twitching of the hands, he may suggest to the subject, "The more your hands twitch, the lighter they become. You can feel the lightness in your hands. They are becoming so light that they are lifting up into the air." If these suggestions are accepted, the operator continues with the induction by arm levitation. The subject may continue to defend himself by becoming so relaxed that his arm lacks sufficient tone to maintain itself in an upright position. If this occurs, the operator should immediately return to suggestions of relaxation. In this way, the subject's defenses are continually exploited until he finally accepts the suggestions and drifts into hypnosis.

In the dynamic method of induction, the next suggestion is always determined by the subject's response to the previous one. The operator always uses the subject's defense in the actual hypnotic induction, and he always changes the suggestions to an area in which the subject's defense is not presently applicable.

The successful use of the dynamic method demands adaptability on the part of the operator. He must always be ready to change the nature of his suggestions according to the subject's defenses, which may vary from moment to moment. The dynamic method is more difficult to learn than any of the other methods, because the operator never knows what the next suggestions will be, since they are determined by the subject's defenses at the moment. The operator must not only be alert to the meaning of the subject's behavior, but also secure in himself, so that there is no chance of his communicating anxiety or a feeling of failure to the subject.

The dynamic method is best with subjects who are difficult to hypnotize. Many subjects who are considered unsuggestible can be hypnotized by the dynamic method, if they have adequate motivation and if a proper rapport between the subject and the hypnotic operator has been established.

THE AUTHORITATIVE DIRECT STARE INDUCTION

This induction technique is of real importance in hypnotherapy. Sometimes it is the only effective means of dealing with a hyperacute anxiety reaction, which takes place when an abreacting client suddenly comes out of hypnosis and becomes aware of previously subconscious traumatic material. If such a situation arises, the authoritative use of the direct stare may be the only effective way of rehypnotizing the subject.

The client may be in any position—standing, sitting or lying down. If standing, the subject should be placed immediately in front of an easy chair so that as he becomes hypnotized, he can be told that his legs can no longer support him and that he will flop down into the chair behind him. Meares (1960) has given an excellent description of this technique.

Following are the steps for the induction of hypnosis by the authoritative direct stare approach:

1. Your head and eyes should be above those of the subject.
2. Command the subject to look into your eyes.
3. The following suggestions should be given loudly, clearly, and with an air of complete command: "You look at me. You look at my eyes. Your eyelids are getting heavier and heavier. You feel the heaviness of your eyelids. They get heavier and heavier. You can't keep them open."
4. The client's eyelids usually blink, or at least flutter. Seize upon this as evidence that he cannot keep them open. Give the following suggestions: "Yes, they blink. You can't keep them

open. Your eyelids are so heavy that you can't keep them open. Your eyelids are heavy and sticky. You feel them sticking down so that you can hardly open them. You are struggling hard to keep them open. It is no good. They are irresistibly heavy. You try to keep them open by raising your eyebrows. But it is no good. The irresistible heaviness is all through them. You can't keep them open."

5. Conclude with the following suggestions: "Your eyes are closing now . . . your eyes are closing . . . they close . . . they are stuck down with heaviness . . . you cannot open them."

In summary: if the client appears to be relaxed, induce hypnosis by the progressive relaxation method; if he appears to be tense, use the arm levitation induction method; if the client is negativistic, induce hypnosis by means of repetitive movement; if the client manifests sustained defenses, employ the dynamic method of induction, and if an abreacting client suddenly comes out of hypnosis, use the authoritative direct stare for quick reinduction of the hypnotic state.

Chapter 7.

Induction Techniques with Children

The three cardinal rules in using hypnosis with children are: (1) gain the child's confidence; (2) tell him what you are going to do, and (3) consider the age and intelligence of the child when choosing the words in the induction technique and in talking to the child.

Techniques of induction applicable to children are varied; selection of the most suitable technique for a particular child can be made only after sufficient experience is acquired by the hypnotic operator. The following have proven to be the most effective techniques with children.

TV TECHNIQUE

This technique is effective with children in the age range from three to nine. It is an effective technique because most children enjoy watching television. The child is asked to close his eyes and to listen to the operator. Then a conversation is started about TV programs and the child's favorite program is determined. He is then asked to imagine a magic TV set which he can turn on and focus. He is then told to find the station for his favorite TV program and to relax and enjoy the show. The operator may check on progress by asking the child from time to time to relate what is going on. The child will usually relate in a very vivid manner what he is seeing on the TV screen.

FALLING BACKWARD

This method is practical for children between six and eight years of age. The child is asked to stand with his arms fully extended and close to his sides, and with his feet close together. The operator tilts the child's head back so that his chin is lifted upward. Then the child is asked to close his eyes and hold his head steady. The operator assures the child that he will not be allowed to fall. Then the child is told that the operator is going to count from one to three, that with each count, he will feel himself falling backward, and that as he is falling backward, he will be getting drowsy. He is also told that as soon as his back touches the couch, he will be completely relaxed. The count should be carried out slowly with the operator's hands on the child's shoulder blades and supporting the body. The falling should be continued to about a 45-degree angle and then the child is lifted bodily and placed lying on his back on the couch. Suggestions of being comfortable and relaxed are continued.

MODIFIED HAND LEVITATION

This method is easily applied to children from nine to twelve years of age. The child should be seated on a chair with the operator directly in front of him. Then the child is asked to place his hands on his lap with the palms facing down. An ink spot is placed on the knuckle of the right index finger and the child is asked to focus his gaze on the spot. Then the operator places his hands on the hands of the child, exerting pressure on the child's hands and suggesting that they are getting heavier and heavier. As the pressure is gradually slackened, the child is told that his hands are feeling lighter and lighter and will float up into the air. He is told that he will watch the ink spot come closer and closer to his face and that as soon as any part of his hands touch his face, his hands will fall limply into his lap, his eyes will close and he will become deeply relaxed.

EYE FIXATION WITH PROGRESSIVE RELAXATION

This method is frequently successful with the older child. The child is seated and asked to take a deep breath, hold it for several seconds, then exhale slowly and concentrate on letting all of his muscles relax completely as he exhales. This is repeated and then the child is asked to place his hands on his lap, palms down. The ink spot is used as in the modified hand levitation method. The child is told to focus his gaze on the spot and then the operator proceeds with progressive relaxation of each muscle group, beginning with the forehead, then the face muscles, the neck muscles, the shoulders, the arms, hands and fingers, the back muscles, the stomach muscles and the legs, feet and toes. A slight pause should be made after suggestions of relaxation of each muscle group. Then the suggestion is given that as the whole body remains relaxed and as he keeps his gaze on the ink spot, his eyelids will get heavier and heavier; the suggestion is then made that his eyes will close and that as soon as they close, he will be deeply relaxed and will continue to go deeper and deeper relaxed.

Eye Fixation on Egg Timer

This method of induction is quite suitable for young children. A three-minute hourglass type of egg timer is most suitable. The child is told that the sand in the glass is magic sand obtained from the Sandman. He is told that as he watches the sand fall from the top of the glass to the bottom, he will become very sleepy and that he will have dropped off to sleep by the time all of the sand has fallen to the bottom of the glass, but that he will still be able to hear what the operator is saying to him. The egg timer is then placed where the child can watch it and additional suggestions of drowsiness and sleep are given as the child watches the falling sand.

Sleepy Animal Technique

This technique can be used very effectively with young children, especially a recalcitrant two- or three-year-old. The operator should have the child's mother bring the child's favorite toy animal along to the treatment session. Then, when the child is seated and holding the toy animal, he should be told that the animal is now going to sleep. Then the child is told that he had better be quiet, or he might wake the animal (refer to the animal by name if it has one). The child should then be told that he can see that the animal's leg is loose. The operator should then pick up the leg of the toy and let it loose. Then he should pick up the other leg and let it fall down in a relaxed way, pick up the animal's floppy ear and let it fall down, and so on. Then the child should be told to be very careful to let the animal sleep. In the process of helping the toy animal to sleep, the child gets very relaxed and very often will go into a light state of hypnosis. Although a two- or three-year-old child will not exhibit a large range of hypnotic phenomena, he can show such phenomena as restricted awareness, catalepsy, and anesthesia.

AMBROSE'S INDUCTION METHOD WITH CHILDREN

Dr. Gordon Ambrose (1961: 38-39) reported a method that he found to be very satisfactory with children. The child is placed in a comfortable armchair and is immediately told to relax and loosen all of his muscles. He is then asked if he is warm and comfortable. The room is darkened and the following words are used:

"Now you feel very comfortable, very calm; I want you to look at this light, as you look at the light you will feel your muscles beginning to get loose. You feel lovely and warm and comfortable. You will remember everything that happens. When I tell you, you will become very drowsy, very heavy, and very sleepy. Now you look at the light, your eyes are getting heavy, very heavy, they want to close. Close your eyes—now!!!

The word *NOW* is emphasized. The operator stands in front of the child holding the light in his right hand, with his left arm raised and bent at the elbow with the palm facing outwards. As the child looks at the light and the directions are given—"Your eyes are heavy, they close now"—on the word *now*, the fingers on the left hand are slightly bent and the arm then falls to the side in almost the same movement. When the child's eyes close, the following suggestions are given:

"You are becoming drowsy and heavy and sleepy. The more you listen to my voice, the deeper, the more drowsy, the more sleepy you become. You are feeling lovely and comfortable; calm and drowsy, deeper and deeper asleep. You will listen to every word I say. As you become more and more drowsy, you will feel more and more happy. You will feel a sense of calmness and happiness, all your limbs are lovely and loose; you feel more and more drowsy and sleepy. Now I will count slowly to five. As I begin to count, you will feel more and more sleepy, more and more drowsy, until I reach the number five. As I say *five* you will go into a very deep, drowsy, sleepy state, listening to every word I say."

The operator counts slowly to five, emphasizing the number when he reaches it.

TWO-FINGER EYE-CLOSURE METHOD

This method is described by Elman (1964: 41-42). The following excerpt from Elman's book is a good description of this method.

Jean, I guess you play a lot with your dolls when you're home. And you probably pretend a lot with them, isn't that right? Well, we have a little game of pretend too. And if you can learn to play this little game of pretend, nothing that happens in the dentist's office will bother or disturb you. You just won't feel anything that we're doing if you learn to play this little game. Would you like to learn it? [Patient answers yes]. All right, open your eyes wide. I'm going to show you this little game. I'm going to pull your eyes shut with my forefinger and my thumb, like this. [Gently places thumb and finger on eyelids and draws them down]. Now you pretend with your whole heart and soul that you can't open your eyes. That's all you have to do. Just pretend that. Now, I will take my hand away [removes hand] and you pretend so hard that when you try to open your eyes they just won't work. Now try to make them work while you're pretending. Try hard. They just won't work, see. Now just because you're pretending like that, anything we do in this office won't bother or disturb you at all. In your mind you can be home playing with your dolls and you won't feel anything I have to do.

"Magic" Doll Technique

The doctor or dentist has a doll in his office and tells his small patient that it is a magic doll and that as long as he is holding the magic doll he won't feel anything. This is an effective method for achieving hypnoanesthesia in young children.

"Magic Circle" Technique

This method is also effective for achieving hypnoanesthesia in young children. The doctor or nurse draws a circle on the child's arm in the area where he is to be given a shot. The child is told that this is a magic circle, and that he will not feel anything within that circle.

"Magic" Medicine Technique

This is a placebo method. It is most effective with children between the ages of three and seven. The child is told that the doctor has some very special magic medicine: whenever anybody takes some of the magic medicine, they get very sleepy and in a short time they close their eyes and have a very nice dream. Then the child is given a dose of the magic medicine (colored water), with accompanying suggestions of drowsiness.

On-Off Switch Technique for Achieving Hypnoanesthesia in Children

This method requires that the child be old enough to comprehend the concept of the conduction of electricity through wires. The child is told that we have wires in the body that connect to switches in the head. When the switches in the head are on, we feel pain; when they are off, we don't feel pain. Then the child is told to close his eyes and to pretend that his right thumb is transparent, that he can see through it. Then he is asked to tell the color of the wire. He is then asked to pretend that his arm from the thumb to the elbow is transparent and that he can see the wire all the way to the elbow. Then he is asked to pretend that the part of his body from the elbow to the neck is transparent and that he can see the wire all the way to the neck.

He is told that now he can see the wire connected to a little box in the middle of his head. He is then told that there are some switches on one side of the box and asked to tell on which side the switches are. Then he is asked how many switches there are. When he responds, he is told that all of the switches are the same color except one. Then he is asked to give the color of the majority of the switches and the color of the different one. Then he is told to mentally reach up and turn off the electricity to his right arm and hand and that any pain to that arm and hand is now turned off. He is told that the left hand is still connected and that it can still feel pain (test with sharp instrument to convince child). He is then told that he can feel the right hand but that he cannot feel any pain in it (test for anesthesia).

Finally, he is told that anything he touches with the disconnected hand will also become disconnected. Then have the child demonstrate his ability to shut off the pain in various parts of his body.

Part Three
Stages of Hypnosis and Recognition of Depth

Chapter 8.

Recognition of the Depth of the Hypnotic State: Clinical Depth Scales

All investigators have been led to the conclusion that hypnosis occurs in degrees. However, there is no general agreement concerning the number of hypnotic stages, nor is there any agreement concerning the objective symptoms or phenomena included within each stage. It is difficult to objectively determine where one of the various stages ends and another begins. However, the hypnotic operator with adequate training and a sufficient amount of experience can usually make a close approximation.

For teaching purposes, six divisions of the various stages of hypnosis are sufficient. The first four of these are sufficient for most clinical purposes.

1. Hypnoidal—the lightest recognizable level; precursor to hypnosis
2. Light stage
3. Medium stage
4. Somnambulism—necessary for reconstructive hypnoanalysis
5. Coma or plenary stage
6. Hypnosleep—hypnosis attached to sleep

The clinical depth scales to be presented in this chapter are quantitative scales. These are good as a reference standard in a clinical setting but they lack specificity with respect to induction techniques and quantification of response, thus making them unsatisfactory as psychometric research instruments.

Some of the scales for measuring depth of hypnosis are included in Tables 1 through 5. The objective symptoms will generally manifest themselves at the same level of depth for each subject, but not necessarily in the same sequence. Depth should not be determined on the basis of an isolated objective symptom, but rather on the manifestation of at least several symptoms at the particular level of depth.

TABLE 1.
DAVIS-HUSBAND SCALE (1931)

Depth	Objective Symptoms
Insusceptible	0
Hypnoidal	1 Relaxation 2 Fluttering of lids 3 Closing of eyes 4 Complete physical relaxation
Light trance	5 Catalepsy of eyes 6 Limb catalepsy 7 Rigid catalepsy 8 Anesthesia (glove)
Medium trance	9 Partial amnesia 10 Posthypnotic anesthesia 11 Personality changes 12 Simple posthypnotic suggestions 13 Kinesthetic delusions; complete amnesia
Somnambulistic trance	14 Ability to open eyes without affecting trance 15 Bizarre posthypnotic suggestions 16 Complete somnambulism 17 Positive visual hallucinations, posthypnotic 18 Positive auditory hallucinations, posthypnotic 19 Systematized posthypnotic amnesias 20 Negative auditory hallucinations 21 Negative visual hallucinations; hyperesthesias

TABLE 2.
LE CRON-BORDEAUX SCALE (1947)

Depth	Objective Symptoms
Insusceptible	0
Hypnoidal	1 Physical relaxation 2 Drowsiness apparent 3 Fluttering of eyelids 4 Closing of eyes 5 Mental relaxation, partial lethargy of mind 6 Heaviness of limbs
Light trance	7 Catalepsy of eyes 8 Partial limb catalepsy 9 Inhibition of small muscle groups 10 Slower and deeper breathing, slower pulse 11 Strong lassitude (disinclination to move, speak, think or act) 12 Twitching of mouth or jaw during induction 13 Rapport between subject and operator 14 Simple posthypnotic suggestions 15 Involuntary start or eye twitch on awakening 16 Personality changes 17 Feeling of heaviness throughout entire body 18 Partial feeling of detachment
Medium trance	19 Recognition of trance 20 Complete muscular inhibitions (kinesthetic illusions) 21 Partial amnesia

TABLE 2.
LeCron-Bordeaux Scale (1947)—(Continued)

Depth	Objective Symptoms
	22 Glove anesthesia
	23 Tactile illusions
	24 Gustatory illusions
	25 Olfactory illusions
	26 Hyperacuity to atmospheric conditions
	27 Complete catalepsy of limbs or body
Deep or somnambulistic trance	28 Ability to open eyes without affecting trance
	29 Fixed stare when eyes are open; pupillary dilation
	30 Somnambulism
	31 Complete amnesia
	32 Systematized posthypnotic amnesias
	33 Complete anesthesia
	34 Posthypnotic anesthesia
	35 Bizarre posthypnotic suggestions
	36 Uncontrolled movement of eyeballs
	37 Detached feeling
	38 Rigidity and lag in muscular movements
	39 Fading and increase in cycles of sound of operator's voice
	40 Control of organic body functions
	41 Hypermnesia
	42 Age regression
	43 Positive visual hallucinations
	44 Negative visual hallucinations

TABLE 2.
LeCron-Bordeaux Scale (1947)—(Continued)

Depth	Objective Symptoms
	45 Positive auditory hallucinations 46 Negative auditory hallucinations 47 Stimulation of dreams 48 Hyperasthesias 49 Color sensations experienced
Plenary trance	50 Stuporous condition in which all spontaneous activity is inhibited

TABLE 3.
HERON DEPTH SCALE (1957)

Depth	Objective Symptoms
Insusceptible	0 No response to suggestion other than that one would get from the average individual in the waking state
Hypnoidal	1 Relaxation 2 Fluttering and closing of eyelids if eye fixation techniques are used 3 Profound physical relaxation
Light	4 Catalepsy of eyes 5 Limb catalepsy
Medium	6 Simple motor reaction without awakening 7 Simple posthypnotic suggestion 8 Glove anesthesia 9 Amnesia 10 Posthypnotic anesthesia 11 Extend verbal discourse without awakening
Deep	12 Ability to open eyes without it affecting the hypnotic state 13 Positive hallucinations 14 Negative hallucinations

TABLE 4.
ARONS MASTER DEPTH RULE (1961)

Depth	Stage	Objective
Light	1	1 Lethargy 2 Relaxation 3 Eye Catalepsy
Light	2	4 Catalepsy of isolated muscle groups 5 Heavy or floating feelings
Medium	3	6 Rapport 7 Smell and taste changes 8 Number block (aphasia)
Medium	4	9 Amnesia—also posthypnotic 10 Analgesia 11 Automatic movements
Somnambulism	5	12 Positive hallucinations 13 Bizarre posthypnotic suggestions
Somnambulism	6	14 Negative hallucinations 15 Plenary or comatose trance via suggestion

TABLE 5.
HARTMAN DEPTH SCALE (1968)

Depth	Objective Symptoms
Insusceptible	0 No response to suggestion other than that one would get from individual in waking state
Hypnoidal	1 Body warmth 2 Dilation of pupils 3 Increased lacrimation 4 Whites of eyes getting red or pink 5 Blinking and involuntary drooping of eyelids 6 Eye closure 7 Partial physical relaxation
Light Depth	8 Eyelid catalepsy 9 Partial limb catalepsy (lifted limb remains upright but slowly falls) 10 Breathing becomes slower, but is still shallow, diaphragmatic 11 Slowing of muscular activity
Medium Depth	12 Complete physical relaxation 13 Breathing becomes deeper and more regular 14 Some loss of motor activity 15 Glove analgesia 16 Loss of interest in extraneous environmental sounds 17 Partial amnesia 18 Simple posthypnotic suggestion 19 Marked limb catalepsy 20 Glove anesthesia 21 Posthypnotic analgesia

TABLE 5.

Hartman Depth Scale (1968)—(Continued)

Depth	Objective Symptoms
	22 Increased concentration on words of operator
Artificial somnambulism	23 Aphasia (subject unwilling to articulate numbers but hasn't forgotten them)
Somnambulism	24 Ability to open eyes without affecting trance
	25 Complete amnesia (artificial)
	26 Anesthesia of any part of the body (with suggestion)
	27 Posthypnotic anesthesia
	28 Bizarre posthypnotic suggestions
	29 Feeling of detachment
	30 Fading in and out of operator's voice
	31 Control of autonomic nervous system functions (heartbeat, blood pressure, etc.)
	32 Control of reflexes (with suggestion—knee jerk, patellar reflex, etc.)
	33 Hyperesthesia
	34 Hypermnesia
	35 Age regression and revivification
	36 Positive gustatory and olfactory hallucinations
	37 Positive visual hallucinations
	38 Positive auditory hallucinations
	39 Negative gustatory and olfactory hallucinations
	40 Negative visual hallucinations
	41 Negative auditory hallucinations
	42 Stimulation of dreams

TABLE 5.
Hartman Depth Scale (1968)—(Continued)

Depth	Objective Symptoms
Coma or Plenary State	43 Inhibition of all spontaneous activity 44 Feeling of euphoria 45 Anesthesia without suggestion 46 Inability to move a large group of muscles (i.e., arm or leg) 47 Inability to move a small group of muscles such as those around the eyes (no movement whatsoever) 48 Catatonia without suggestion
Hypnosleep	49 True amnesia 50 Lack of conscious awareness

Chapter 9.

The Coma State: How to Induce It, How to Test for It and How to Use It

Although a light or medium stage of hypnosis is suitable for purposes of physical relaxation and hypnotic suggestions for ego strengthening, desensitization and other methods of symptom removal, somnambulism is essential for most types of hypnoanalytic work. Therefore, the hypnotic operator should know how to achieve this state. Chapter Twenty-six gives a verbatim detailed account of how to achieve somnambulism; if all of the steps are followed precisely, the majority of subjects will be capable of achieving somnambulism.

This chapter will be devoted to a stage of hypnosis that has received very little attention, and, consequently, many hypnotic operators have panicked when a subject hasn't come out of hypnosis when asked to or hasn't responded to questions. If the operators had been aware of the coma state, there would have been no cause for alarm.

The coma or plenary state is an even deeper state of hypnosis than somnambulism. Dave Elman (1964) developed an excellent method for achieving the coma state, testing for it, and arousing the subject from it. Every hypnotic operator should be aware of the coma state, know how to induce it, how to test for it and how to use it. There is never any danger that the subject will not come out of the coma state.

The coma state brings with it a complete euphoria. In this state, nothing bothers or disturbs the subject. Also, the subject is able to give himself a complete anesthesia. Although the subject will not respond either verbally or nonverbally in the coma state, he has complete awareness: when questioned after having been in the coma state, he can relate everything that occurred.

The following steps should be followed in order to achieve and test for the coma state.

1. First, get the subject into the somnambulistic state.

2. Use the elevator-deepening technique to get the subject down to the "basement of relaxation." The following procedure was developed by Dave Elman to induce the coma state:

> I know how relaxed you are, but even in your relaxed state, I'll bet you sense in your own mind that there is a state of relaxation below the one you're in right now. Can you sense that? . . . You know that you can clench your fist and make it tighter and tighter and tighter—and you might call that the height of tension. You can relax that same fist until you can't relax it any more. You might call that the basement of relaxation. I'm going to try to take you down to the basement. . . . To get down to floor A, you have to relax twice as much as you have relaxed already. To get down to floor B, you have to relax twice as much as you did at floor A, and to get down to C, you have to relax twice as much as you did at floor B. But when you reach floor C, that is the basement of relaxation, and at that point you will give off signs by which I will be able to tell that you are at the basement. You don't know what these signs are, and I'm not going to tell you what they are, but every person who has ever been at the basement of relaxation gives off those signs. . . . You will ride down to floor A on an imaginary elevator and you will use that same elevator to get down to the basement of relaxation. You are on that elevator now. When I snap my fingers, that elevator will start down. If you relax twice as much as you have relaxed already, you will be down at floor A. Tell me when you are at floor A by saying the letter A out loud.

Follow the same procedure to take the subject down to floor B and then floor C, the basement of relaxation.

3. Then, without a word of suggestion, proceed to give the first test for the coma state—a test for anesthesia.

4. Then ask the subject to try to move a large group of muscles, such as an arm or a leg. If the subject doesn't respond, the second test for the coma state has been successful.

5. Then ask the subject to open his eyes. In the true coma state, there is no movement of the eyeballs or eyelids whatsoever.

6. The fourth and final test is for limb catalepsy without suggestion. Place an arm or leg in a certain position; if the subject is in the coma state, it will remain in that position.

If the subject is in a true coma state, he cannot be aroused by ordinary means. We know that the subject is in a state of euphoria when in the hypnotic coma and is reluctant to give up this wonderful feeling. The best way to bring the subject out of the coma state is to threaten to deprive him of his euphoria by telling him that if he doesn't come out of hypnosis on a given signal, he will never again be able to experience the wonderful state he is now in. With this possibility in mind, the subject will find it easy to open his eyes when instructed to do so.

The coma state has many uses. To mention only a few: in arthritis and cancer patients, to relieve intractible pain; in postoperative procedures, particularly when the patient must be immobilized in a particular position for an extended period of time; in surgery—physicians have reported using the coma state for nose and throat operations, brain surgery, heart surgery, hysterectomy, appendectomy, reduction of compound fractures and many other kinds of operations; and in obstetrics, during actual childbirth.

Chapter 10.

Hypnosleep: Hypnosis Attached to Sleep

Once a person is asleep, it is reasonably easy to attach hypnosis to his sleep state. When this is done, the deepest hypnotic state possible will be secured. In any other state of hypnosis, even in the coma state, the subject has complete awareness. But when he is hypnotized in his sleep, he usually has no recollection whatever upon awakening, and usually the amnesia cannot be completely removed. When amnesia is encountered in any other state of hypnosis, even in the coma state, it can be completely removed by suggestion. The amnesia that occurs in somnambulism is a false amnesia and can be removed at will. However, when the hypnotic state is attached to sleep, the amnesia is deep. Even when prodded, the subject does not have total recall.

There are many potential uses for this deepest state of hypnosis. Extremely powerful anesthesia can be given; preoperative tension and anxiety can be completely removed, and psychotherapists have stated that with this technique, they have the perfect device for probing into the subconscious mind of the patient who has the memory of traumatic events buried deeply below the level of conscious awareness.

The following steps, which have been formulated by Elman (1964), are necessary in order to obtain the hypnosleep state:

1. Count the number of respirations per minute while the subject is fully awake. [A healthy person during his waking hours breathes at the rate of sixteen to eighteen times per minute.]
2. Put the subject into somnambulism.

3. Give the subject sleep suggestions to take effect on cue, after he is aroused from the hypnotic state.

4. Arouse the subject from the hypnotic state and then let him go into a natural sleep state on cue.

5. Count the respirations of the subject. Make sure breathing is down to six or seven times a minute. If the subject is breathing too fast, wait until he is more soundly asleep.

6. The purpose is to bypass the critical faculty without awakening the subject; therefore, the hypnotic operator should approach the subject very gently and say the following in a soft but confident tone of voice: "This is [your name] speaking. You can hear me, but you won't wake up. You can hear me, but you won't wake up."

7. The subject is usually in such a deep sleep that the above must be repeated several times before it penetrates his subconscious mind. Then continue with the following: "I'll know you are hearing me when your right index finger, which I am now touching, begins to rise. I'll know you are hearing me when your right index finger moves. You can hear me, but you won't wake up."

8. When the right index finger rises, continue to talk softly, compounding suggestions as you proceed.

9. When you have finished giving the desired instructions or concluded the hypnoanalysis by means of ideomotor questioning (see Chapter Twenty-seven), your next step is to remove the hypnotic state and return the subject to the natural sleep state. When the hypnosleep state has been induced in the hypnotic operator's office, the client is told that he will sleep for five minutes and then awaken refreshed and relaxed. When hypnosleep is induced during the night, the client is told that he will sleep soundly throughout the night and that in the morning he will awaken, completely refreshed.

Part Four
Types of
Hypnotherapy

Chapter 11.

Hypnoidal Therapy

There are sometimes reasons for not attempting to hypnotize a client, at least in the early stage of therapy. The client may be too insecure to allow himself to go into hypnosis. Prepsychosis or latent homosexuality may contraindicate hypnosis. Such individuals may benefit from hypnoidal therapy.

The hypnoidal state is characterized by complete physical relaxation with an uncritical state of mind. It is a borderline state between the waking state and the actual hypnotic state. As pointed out by Weitzenhoffer (1957), the dreamy condition associated with the hypnoidal state has been found valuable in psychotherapy, and, because of the enhanced suggestibility of the hypnoidized client, it is possible to give a large variety of suggestions successfully. Weitzenhoffer has also stated that it should be kept in mind that there is little evidence for thinking that the hypnoidal state is not a mild state of hypnosis. In discussing the giving of suggestions while the client is in the hypnoidal state, Meares (1960) stated, "Easy suggestions are accepted without question, but a suggestion that carries any difficulty of acceptance is likely to evoke the critical faculties and to bring the patient out of the hypnoidal state to alert consciousness". [p. 275]

There are a number of advantages to the hypnoidal state. One advantage is that it can be induced without reference to hypnosis, a fact of importance in handling difficult or resistant clients or individuals with strong initial misconceptions about hypnosis. Another advantage is that in most cases, it involves a simpler procedure than hypnosis. Also, it is possible to hypnoidize far more individuals than can be hypnotized to any other degree.

The hypnoidal state may be induced in the following manner. First, tell the client that you can help him get rid of tension by showing him how to relax. Then have the client lie on the couch and proceed to induce relaxation, primarily by nonverbal means. Move the client's limbs and allow them to flop, and encourage the relaxation of the abdominal musculature by gentle touch. Give a few slowly spoken suggestions of relaxation simultaneously with the nonverbal means of communication. As soon as the client manifests the signs of being physically relaxed, such as eyelid closure, muscle flaccidity, and deep and regular breathing, then the therapist can proceed with suggestions of calmness.

The client is aroused from the hypnoidal state by the therapist assuming a normal conversational tone of voice. This serves as an extraverbal cue for the client to resume alert consciousness. There is no need to give any countersuggestions to remove the effect of the suggestions to induce the hypnoidal state because the only suggestions that have been given are those of relaxation and calmness.

In many cases, the client develops greater passivity and a greater sense of trust with the therapist after a few sessions of hypnoidal therapy, making it possible to progress to one of the other types of hypnotherapy.

Hypnoidal therapy is indicated with introverts and prepsychotics, for purposes of explanation and persuasion, as an anesthetic during medical office procedures and with individuals who have strong misconceptions about hypnosis. With prepsychotics, hypnosis per se is often contraindicated because of the danger of precipitating an active psychotic process.

Use of Hypnoidal Therapy with Introverts

Because the introvert or schizoid personality has found emotional contact with others so difficult and painful, he defends himself by withdrawal and isolation (rejecting others before they have a chance to reject him). We must respect this defense and must allow our own emotional relationship with him to develop slowly so that it is within the capacity and ego strength of the client to tolerate it. We thus proceed in a leisurely manner, emphasizing relaxation, calmness and inner peace of mind and making judicious use of explanation and persuasion.

USE OF HYPNOIDAL THERAPY WITH PREPSYCHOTICS

In this relationship, the client gains security with the therapist, and by drawing on the ego strength and support of the therapist, it may be possible for him to fend off an impending psychosis through the emotional relationship with the therapist and not in response to any direct suggestions.

USE OF HYPNOIDAL THERAPY FOR EXPLANATION AND PERSUASION

Sometimes hypnoidal therapy can be used for explanation. The client in the hypnoidal state may accept an explanation for his illness that he would reject in the critical state of normal wakefulness. When this technique is used, the hypnoidal state is induced and the therapist talks to the client quietly and slowly. He talks in such a way as to give the client the extraverbal communication to listen and not comment on what is being said. The process involved is not suggestion but persuasion.

Chapter 12.

Direct Hypnotherapy

Direct hypnotherapy is indicated for alleviation of anxiety, alteration of behavior patterns and attitudes and for the removal of symptoms that are not the manifestation of active psychological conflict. Persuasion and reassurance may be incorporated into hypnotherapeutic treatment. These measures are conceptualized within the hypnotherapist's own theoretical frame of reference to some degree.

Active psychological conflict is a contraindication for direct hypnotherapy. If there is active conflict, it should be dealt with by hypnoanalysis. In most cases, symptoms then remit spontaneously. Sometimes, even when relevant conflicts have been worked through in hypnoanalysis, some symptoms persist, and these can be relieved by one of the hypnotherapeutic techniques to be described in this chapter.

Symptoms that are maintained by vicious circle mechanisms are eminently suitable for treatment by direct hypnotherapy. The vicious circle is broken. As there are no active psychological conflicts, there are no complications.

In selecting cases for direct hypnotherapy, we must always assess the degree to which the symptom has become integrated into the personality of the client. The maintenance of the symptom by ongoing or reactivated conflicts, the use of the symptom for secondary gain or the integration of the symptom into the personality are all contraindications for direct symptom removal by hypnotherapy. In suitable cases, the initiating conflict is no longer operative and the symptom is maintained by habit or a vicious circle mechanism. This can be determined by ideomotor questioning during the diagnostic phase of treatment.

In discussing direct symptom removal, Dr. Jerome Schneck (1970) stated:

> Symptoms operating at the periphery of personality functioning can give way to behavioral adaptations and psychological readjustments and such sysmptoms may be relinquished without concern. If compensatory mechanisms come into operation, reappearance of symptoms is unlikely. If these mechanisms are not effective, the symptoms may return or be replaced by others. It is doubtful that the latter is observed as frequently as is claimed by those concerned about it. . . . The idea of symptom removal may give rise to fantasies, among its opponents, of persistent pressuring tactics that entail no respect for degrees of ego strength or weakness. This criticism, when warranted, pertains to therapeutic method and management in general, rather than to hypnotherapy specifically. Usually symptom alleviation moves hand in hand with efforts to strengthen existing personality resources. And this strengthening process is, of course, consistent with aims of treatment in all areas, especially so in the realm of mental health [1970, pp. 22, 23].

Brief descriptions of the specialized hypnotherapeutic techniques available to the hypnotherapist follow:

DIRECT SUGGESTION OF SYMPTOM REMOVAL

This is the oldest and still most widely used of hypnotherapeutic techniques. There is scarcely any functional disturbance that has not been successfully treated by the technique of direct suggestion in hypnosis.

It is highly unlikely that there will be a release of acute anxiety, the appearance of substitute symptoms or a relapse as a result of direct symptom removal, provided that the symptom is not an integral part of the client's personality and that the direct symptom removal is preceded by the regular employment of a sequence of suggestions aimed directly at strengthening the client's ego. I routinely employ the ego-strengthening technique developed by Dr. John Hartland (1965, 1971). The technique is included in the chapter on the second phase of hypnotherapy, the training phase.

As in the induction of hypnosis, there are two different approaches to the removal of symptoms by direct suggestion, the authoritative and the passive. In authoritative symptom removal, the hypnotic operator commands the client to give up the symptom. In passive symptom removal, the hypnotic operator becomes a supportive figure who cajoles the client into abandoning the symptom.

Symptom removal by direct suggestion may take place at a single session, or the symptom may be gradually ameliorated over a number of sessions. The gradual amelioration technique is easier for both therapist and client. It is well suited for subjective symptoms, such as tension and anxiety. It is also valuable in psychosomatic cases.

DIRECTED EXPERIENCE HYPNOTIC TECHNIQUE

With this technique, the client is allowed to experience, under positive affective conditions, situations that had previously aroused anxiety.

The most common behavior therapy technique used for anxiety reduction is systematic desensitization (Wolpe, 1961). The results of an experiment by Gibbons et al. (1970) demonstrated that the Directed Experience Hypnotic Technique (DET) was more effective than systematic desensitization (SD). This is due to a number of factors. First, DET utilizes control of the situation to induce a pleasant affect directly; therefore, the degree of emotional attachment to the test-taking situation involves the totality of the organism as opposed to the selected response elements of SD. Second, DET goes directly to a maximally anxiety-arousing situation, whereas SD uses a hierarchy. Third, DET controls the client's psychological environment, so the client actually believes he is experiencing the suggested situation. With SD, the client imagines the situation, which does not produce as great an intensity of subjective experience. Fourth, DET provides an interpretation of the experience for the client, whereas in SD, the client is left to make his own interpretation.

HYPEREMPIRIA: A TECHNIQUE FOR MIND EXPANSION
AND THE
PRODUCTION OF TRANSPERSONAL PHENOMENA

Hyperempiria is a word coined by Dr. Don Gibbons (1972a, 1972b, 1973, 1974) to denote a greater or enhanced quality of experience. Certain types of experiences, according to Gibbons, are universally meaningful, in that they deal with the central concerns of human existence: time, life, death, God, and the bounds of one's identity and awareness. Transpersonal phenomena such as these are easily induced in a subject who has undergone a previous induction procedure. The subjective reality and esthetic qualities of the experiences are greatly enhanced by a hyperempiric induction based upon suggestions of increased alertness, mind expansion, and enhanced awareness and sensitivity.

Following is a hyperempiric induction procedure (Gibbons, 1972b):

> You are now going to enter a new and different state of awareness called hyperempiria . . . You will find that you begin to experience very pleasant feelings of increased alertness and sensitivity . . . You are beginning to enter into a higher level of consciousness, now, one in which your ability to realize your full capacity for experience is greatly increased—yet you experience no strain or discomfort. Instead, you are feeling a quiet exultation in your ability to use your consciousness so much more effectively. Your range of awareness is pleasantly expanding, and your perceptual abilities are becoming infinitely keener.
>
> As your consciousness expands more and more, you are not experiencing an overloaded awareness, but instead, you feel an inner sense of quiet joy as you come to experience all of your perceptual abilities being tuned to their highest pitch . . . It's a pleasant feeling of release and liberation that you are experiencing now, as all of these great untapped potentials become freed for their fullest possible functioning, and it's not fatiguing or tiring in the least.
>
> Now, all of your perceptual abilities will be tuned to their highest possible pitch within just a few seconds, and you will be able to utilize your full capacity for experience.
>
> Now, you are ready.

After the hyperempiric state of consciousness has been induced, the subject is provided with a series of mind expanding and transpersonal experiences and then returned to a normal state of consciousness. The hyperempiric experiences include psychedelic visual and auditory experiences, creative fantasy, achievement imagery, travel through time and space, and various mystical experiences.

The Hyperempiric Affective Experience is presented here as an example of the wording used in the hyperempiric experiences:

> Now I want you to begin to focus your attention upon your body, and upon the sensations that you experience. As you do so, you are beginning to be aware of a number of changes taking place;

you are beginning to experience great feelings of peace, relaxation and tranquility; and with each breath you take, the feelings of peace and tranquility become clearer, and stronger, and more distinct . . . Bathing your entire being in endless waves of boundless, perfect, and infinite peace . . . and it's as if all of the worry, and all of the tension, and all of the anxiety which you have ever felt is being completely driven out now, and replaced by this perfect feeling of infinite peace and tranquility . . . And along with this perfect peace you are experiencing a new sort of strength and vitality. You can feel vast reserves within yourself and vast previously untapped potential . . . And the knowledge of this potential, and the great confidence that it brings will remain with you; and whenever you employ your abilities in a full and efficient manner, it will be a source of deep satisfaction to you, and you will experience very rewarding feelings of pride, achievement, and accomplishment at having been able to perform so efficiently and so well [1972 (b), pp. 9, 10].

The client may be returned from the hyperempiric state to a normal state of consciousness in the following manner (Gibbons, 1974):

In a moment I am going to count backwards from ten to one, and by the time I get to the count of one you will be back in the usual, everyday state of consciousness in which we spend most of our waking lives.

You will be feeling absolutely wonderful: your mind will be clear and alert, and you will be thrilled and delighted by the pleasant experiences that you have had . . . You will remember everything that has happened, for it will help you to accomplish a great deal of personal growth in the future. But equally important will be your desire to communicate and to share these experiences with others.

And now I will return you to the everyday state of consciousness by counting backwards from ten to one . . . Ten. Coming back now, coming all the way back . . . Nine. Coming down more and more now, and feeling perfectly marvelous as you continue to return . . . Eight . . . Seven . . . Six. Down and down, coming down more and more now . . . Five. Soon you will be all the way down, feeling thrilled and delighted by the pleasant experiences you have had . . . Four . . . Almost back now . . . Three . . . Two . . . Almost back . . . One. You can open your eyes now, feeling wonderful! [p. 53]

THE CONSTRUCTIVE REALISTIC FANTASY

The Constructive Realistic Fantasy is an application of directed fantasy behavior developed by Dr. Abraham Levitsky (1966). In the Constructive Realistic Fantasy (CRF), the client is encouraged to construct and experience selected fantasies, which are designed to be realistic.

One method of applying CRF is to duplicate as far as possible the actual pressures, doubts and anxieties which the client is likely to face in the real life situation. He is instructed to live through in fantasy the kinds of temptations and pressures that he will be faced with—to give full weight to the negative emotional forces that he will be facing.

Another method of applying the CRF technique is to have the client concretize certain ambitions and aspirations that he claims to believe in and to develop an image of what they would really mean in action.

Another application of the CRF technique is to ask the client to imagine what life would be like without the particular symptom in question.

The CRF technique may also be used as a training procedure in problems of interpersonal relations. A client who has repressed anger in a particular situation may be asked to relive that situation in fantasy and behave as he really would have liked to have behaved.

The client frequently acknowledges the need for behavior change but finds it difficult to imagine himself behaving in new ways. He may not be aware of alternative ways of behaving, or even if he is aware of alternatives, his resistance to practicing the new behavior is great. He is therefore asked to practice in fantasy before actual practice of the new behavior.

The usefulness of the CRF technique is based on the following premises:

1. The client will sometimes have no concept of alternatives to his behavior and may require active help in the development of such concepts.

2. The deliberate effort of the client to fantasize desired realistic behavior can help bring to light some of his unconscious resistances and anxieties.

3. The client's early efforts to develop more satisfying concepts will frequently contain elements of the former unrealistic fantasy and bear careful investigation.

4. Encouraging the client to develop a realistic fantasy will help him take steps in the direction of self-change.

5. The CRF technique makes efforts to have the client incorporate into the realistic fantasy a variety of frustrating and anxiety-producing situations for the purpose of trying to insure that the client's development concept takes due account of the limiting and frustrating conditions he is likely to encounter.

HYPNOTIC AVERSIVE CONDITIONING

This is one of the oldest hypnotherapeutic techniques, dating back to the nineteenth century. It has been used to treat compulsive eaters, cigarette smokers, drug addicts and alcoholics. Wolberg (1948) employed the association of painful and disgusting experiences from the client's own life with the undesirable behavior and combines these with associations with hypnotically induced disagreeable fantasies. Erickson (1954b) presented a case of the indirect use of hypnosis of an enuretic married couple which involved a subtle use of aversive conditioning as part of the overall treatment. The following instructions were given to the couple:

> This is what you are to do: Each evening you are to take fluids freely. Two hours before you go to bed, lock the bathroom door after drinking a glass of water. At bedtime, get into your pajamas and then kneel side by side on the bed, facing your pillows and deliberately, intentionally and jointly wet the bed. This may be hard to do, but you must do it. Then lie down and go to sleep, knowing full well that the wetting of the bed is over and done with for the night, that nothing can really make it noticeably wetter. Do this every night, no matter how much you hate it—you have promised, though you did not know what the promise entailed, but you are obligated. Do it every night for two weeks, that is, until Sunday the 17th. On Sunday night, you may take a rest from this task. You may that night lie down and go to sleep in a dry bed. On Monday morning, the 18th, you will arise, throw back the covers, look at the bed. Only as you see a wet bed, then and only then will you realize that there will be before you another three weeks of kneeling and wetting the bed. You have your instructions. There is to be no discussion and no debating between you about this, just silence. There is to be only obedience, and you will then give me a full and amazing account. Goodby! [p. 172]

Five weeks later, the couple returned to Dr. Erickson and reported that they desperately dreaded each night of the first two weeks and looked forward with an increasing intensity of desire to lying down and sleeping in a dry bed on Sunday the 17th. On the morning of Monday the 18th, they were amazed to find the bed still dry. That night they "sneaked" into bed wondering why they had not deliberately wet the bed but at the same time enjoying the comfort of a dry bed. On Tuesday morning, the bed was dry again. That night and thereafter, Monday night's behavior had been repeated.

Kroger (1963) gave the following aversive suggestions to the hypnotized alcoholic patient:

> Each time that you even think of drinking, you will develop a horrible disgust and taste for the liquor by associating it with the most horrible, repugnant smell and taste that you have ever experienced. After you have said this to yourself again and again, you will really begin to believe that a drink will smell and taste awful. [p. 270]

The following aversive posthypnotic suggestions have been used successfully by Kroger (1963) on many smokers:

> If you are really interested in giving up this habit, allow several cigarette butts to remain in the ash tray until they develop a very stale odor. Then sniff this odoriferous ash tray at least once every hour. If you do this, you will easily develop a distaste for cigarettes. May I suggest that another ash tray with stale butts be placed on your night stand beside your bed just before retiring. When you can no longer bear the obnoxious smell, place the ash tray out in the hall, as you should repeat this procedure the next night until every fresh cigarette reminds you of a stale one. [p. 275]

Kroger (1963) has found the following aversive posthypnotic suggestion applicable to most obese patients:

> You might like to think of the most horrible, nauseating and repugnant smell that you have ever experienced. Perhaps it might be the vile odor of rotten eggs. In the future, whenever you desire to eat something that is not on your diet, you will immediately associate this disagreeable smell with it. Also, you might like to think of the most awful and disgusting taste that you may have had in the past. This, too, can be linked up with fattening foods even when you merely think of them. [p. 175]

PSEUDO-ORIENTATION IN TIME

This technique, as described by Erickson (1954a), consists of guiding the hypnotized subject into a dissociated state, in which he believes he has already accomplished something that he previously felt was beyond his ability to achieve.

This technique may be utilized to create a situation in which the client can effectively respond psychologically to desired therapeutic goals as actualities already achieved. As an example of this technique, Erickson (1954a) reported the case of a client suffering from a compulsion to visit his mother's grave every day. This compulsion severely interfered with his life. Erickson had the hypnotized subject project himself two weeks into the future, at which time it was suggested that he fantasize himself to have failed to make his habitual visits to the grave. He was then reoriented to the present, amnesia was suggested for the hypnotic session, and he was brought out of hypnosis and given an appointment two weeks later. During that period he neither visited the grave nor gave it a thought. A follow-up ten years later showed that the compulsion remained abated.

According to Yanovski (1972), the following conditions are essential for the successful utilization of this technique: (1) that the patient perceive the "accomplished" experience as a reality during the trance; (2) that the patient have as complete an amnesia as possible about events leading up to the trance state, and (3) that the therapeutic procedure be based on fantasies that are reasonably realistic to the patient and represent consciously acceptable intentions of the rational part of his ego.

PROLONGED HYPNOSIS

The patient is hypnotized as deeply as possible and is allowed to remain in hypnosis for an extended period, much as in prolonged narcosis. This hypnotherapeutic technique was employed extensively by Wetterstrand (1902), a Swedish hypnotherapist, who frequently kept his patients in deep hypnosis for several days. He likened the therapeutic effect of prolonged hypnosis to the healing power of deep sleep.

This technique is not widely used because of the practical difficulties involved. It may be applied successfully in a hospital situation, where adequate medical and nursing care is available. One such case has been reported in detail by Edwin Baron (1958). The case was that of a 26-year-old mother of three children who was extremely nervous. She was underweight because she couldn't stimulate her appetite, and she suffered from insomnia, which limited her sleep to less than two hours a night. She also had a psychosomatic rash on her left hand. She explained her predicament in this manner: "I'm running in a vicious circle of sleeping pills to knock me out and pep pills to help me keep up with my children." She volunteered for a five-day experiment in prolonged hypnosis after her personal physician gave his approval.

Roughly, this was what the hypnotic operator set out to accomplish:

1. Determine whether a person could actually be kept in hypnosis for five days.
2. Determine whether suggestions given in prolonged hypnosis would have more effect than the traditional type of treatment, when a person would be hypnotized for from 30 minutes to an hour, once or twice a week.
3. Determine what effect prolonged hypnosis had on the psychological, mental and physical condition of the patient.

Three physicians assisted with the experiment. One or more of them examined the patient daily and a graduate nurse supervised a corps of nurses who were with the patient every minute of the five days. To detect any physiological changes which might occur in the patient, she was given basal metabolism tests and EKG, pulse rate and blood pressure examinations before, during and after the experiment. Prior to being put into hypnosis, the patient was given the Rorschach Ink Blot Test which indicated that she had marked emotional instability.

The patient was placed in a specially prepared room and slept continuously 24 hours every day, leaving her bed, still in hypnosis, to eat, wash and be escorted to the bathroom. Since she was underweight, she was put on an especially high calorie diet. Although she had lacked an appetite prior to the experiment, she ate all of the food that was placed before her during the five-day hypnotic hibernation.

At regular intervals, the patient was given the following suggestions:

1. That she would be able to control her emotions and deal with her problems in a rational manner.
2. That she would be tired at night and would be able to get her full eight hours sleep every night.
3. That the rash on her left hand was caused by an emotional

disturbance and that it was getting well and would disappear forever.
4. That she would have an increased appetite and would put on needed weight.
5. That she would no longer be hypersensitive to others touching her.

When the patient came out of the five-day hypnotic state, her first words were, "Well, when do we start? I thought I came up here to go to sleep." It took her several minutes to grasp that the day was Saturday instead of the previous Monday. She became convinced only after she looked closely at her left hand and saw that the rash had disappeared. Physically, her body obtained good rest during the five-day hibernation and she gained four and one-half pounds.

The patient held a news conference one month after the prolonged hypnosis experiment and appeared completely at ease. She told newsmen that many of the things that irritated her before the treatment no longer bothered her. She also reported that she was sleeping normally and had added two more pounds because of her newfound appetite. Also, there was no reappearance of the rash.

Kuriyama (1968) described the following four methods of prolonged hypnosis:

1. Short-term prolonged hypnosis: maintaining the trance for two or three hours.
2. All-night prolonged hypnosis: hypnotizing the patient at night and maintaining the trance, with which the patient goes into natural sleep, until the following morning when he wakes up from hypnosis after washing his face.
3. All-day prolonged hypnosis: maintaining the trance as long as possible on the second day following the all-night hypnosis.
4. Long-term prolonged hypnosis: maintaining the trance all day long, and, moreover, preserving it as long as the subject wishes; if necessary, continuing it for a few days or even for several weeks.

Prolonged hypnosis, according to Kuriyama, is applicable to all cases where hypnotherapy is indicated, but it is of particular use in the following cases:

1. Bronchial asthma, organ neurosis and anxiety neurosis, in which attacks occur every day, particularly during the night.
2. Angina pectoris—chronic stomach ulcer—in which no immediate psychogenic factors are detectable, and where a good

balance of mind and body seems to play an important role in bringing out favorable therapeutic outcomes.

3. Cases of chronic anxiety or tension and those when psychosomatic symptoms are perpetuated.

4. Cases in which no effect can be expected by drug therapy or ordinary hypnotherapy.

Abreaction in Hypnotherapy

The main use of abreaction in hypnotherapy is in symptom removal. The hypnotherapist must keep in emotional contact with the hypnotized client and depth of hypnosis must be maintained.

Abreaction may be induced by giving suggestions that increasingly concern the client's feelings. Suggestions may focus on the client's feelings about his symptom or his feelings about some conflict. When the client shows signs of mounting emotion, such as increased rate and volume of breathing, pallor or flushing of the skin, drawn lips, fixed and watery eyes, restless movements of the arms, and grimacing or nervous twitching of the facial muscles, this emotion can be catalyzed to full-blown abreaction by the hypnotherapist himself entering into the expression of the emotion with the client.

In addition to symptom removal, abreaction is also of value in hypnotherapy of clients with a great deal of tension or aggression. The abreaction allows a return of psychic homeostasis.

Writing Techniques in Hypnotherapy

Coulton (1966) discussed a variety of ways in which writing may be utilized in therapy. First, it can be used as an adjunctive aid in history taking, instructing the patient to write down everything he considers pertinent to his problems and symptoms. Secondly, writing can be used as a rapid method of establishing a correlation between symptoms and emotional states, recurrent situations, interpersonal relationships, or time intervals. Thirdly, writing can be utilized as an uncovering technique. When used in this way, doodling, underlining, misspellings, sudden changes in heaviness or size of the writing and pertinent omissions are often the significant clues. These may be specifically stimulated by hypnotic suggestion. Suggestions may be given to draw or doodle while thinking about the problem, or to draw a picture of how the symptom feels, or to let the hand write or draw in a dissociated state. Fourth, writing can be used as a form of direct therapy. Hypnotic suggestion in conjunction with direct therapy is concerned with stimulating the use of writing as an outlet during times of stress. Emphasis is placed on "getting all the bad feelings out."

> The combination of writing techniques and hypnosis is both natural and helpful. The act of writing often spontaneously produces a hypnoidal state through concentrated attention, exclusion of external stimuli and increased awareness of inner thoughts and feelings. Hypermnesic arousal of associated emotional reactions and time distortion are frequently noted phenomena. Therefore the use of heterohypnosis readily fits this technique. The combined use of these modalities accelerates the therapeutic process. Meaningful material can be reached more rapidly. Psychological blocking is more quickly and versatilely circumvented. Emotional support of the patient is easily accomplished through posthypnotic suggestion. Flexibility in uncovering deeper problems is gained. [Coulton (1966), p. 298]

ATTITUDE THERAPY BY SUGGESTION

Treatment is aimed to correct or improve the basic psychological attitudes of the patient. It is used when the patient's symptoms are found to derive from some faulty attitude or irrational idea.

Attitudes which most commonly concern us are the basic attitudes of masculinity and femininity. In treatment we ignore symptoms which remit spontaneously once we have effected a change in the faulty attitude. A man lacking in masculine assertive drive may present a great variety of symptoms—i.e., feelings of inferiority, premature ejaculation or impotence, etc. These patients can often be helped to greater confidence and to greater self-assertion by hypnosuggestion, using the method of gradual amelioration with attitude and/or rational therapy. Also, the patient may need assertive training in hypnodrama.

The woman patient lacking in feminine passivity may present a great variety of symptoms. Good rapport must be maintained. As little as possible is said about the symptoms, and they gradually subside as the patient develops more feminine basic attitudes. The therapist must remember the theoretical basis of treatment: the aim is to help the patient by suggestion and by the actual experience of passive attitudes in hypnosis. Insight therapy (hypnoanalysis) is to be avoided, as it is likely to arouse both anxiety and aggression in the masculine-aggressive woman; rapport then deteriorates, and chances for successful hypnotherapy are greatly reduced.

Wholesale Desensitization

There are three wholesale desensitization exercises developed by Pierre Clement (1970): The Cloud and the Sun Exercise, the Burning of the Leaves Exercise and the Duck Exercise.

In the Cloud and the Sun Exercise, the client is told to imagine a cloud hovering over and about him. He is then told that his subconscious mind will put into that cloud all that has become a barrier or obstacle to his success in life. Although we don't have to tell the subconscious mind what those obstacles are, we might remind it of a few categories of obstacles: past conditionings such as judgments passed upon us by parents, teachers, friends or neighbors; identification—when we're young we tend to copy and "be like" the people we like, and we copy them so well that we even sometimes copy their shortcomings; guilt—in our subconscious mind we want to punish ourselves for things committed in fact or in imagination and our subconscious mind registers the fact that we shouldn't obtain success "because" we did such things.

At this point, the client is told that we want all of the obstacles to his success in life to be in that cloud, because as he looks at it closely, he will soon detect a source of light somewhere behind or beyond the cloud. When he does see some light he is to let the hypnotic operator know by lifting the index finger of his right hand.

The source of light, the client is told, is really the sun of his own aspirations to be free from those obstacles, the sun of his desires to live a more abundant life. It is then suggested that as the sun becomes brighter and brighter, the client can see the sun's rays make the cloud lift and evaporate and that when the cloud is completely gone, he will be basking in the light of the sun and that he feels its warmth and strength filling him with enthusiasm and certainty.

In the Burning of the Leaves Exercise, the client is told to visualize a garden covered with dried leaves, then to imagine that he finds a rake and sees himself use the rake to pile the many leaves up, finally setting fire to them and stamping them underfoot. The leaves symbolize all the humiliations, all the rebuttals, all the reverses and all the negative conditionings of the client's past life.

The imaginary garden is the garden of his life. When he has gone around a few times to rake up all of the leaves and burn them, he then starts preparing the landscaping of the garden—the bushes, the flower beds, the fountains, etc.

The client is told that the garden can become a mental "retreat," where he can retire anytime he wants to recharge himself and that each time he does the exercise, there will be less and less burning to be done and more and more ornamentation.

The Duck Exercise is a tolerance-of-stress exercise. The client is told to visualize himself in a park, sitting on a bench, under a huge tree, facing a pond where there is a fountain. There are ducks in the pond enjoying the sunshine, plunging their heads into the water and letting the water roll off their backs. Across the pond people are walking about. Suddenly, there comes a downpour, and everybody runs for shelter except the client, who is protected by the huge tree, and the ducks. The ducks just keep paddling along, letting the rain roll off their backs and enjoying the rain just as much as they were previously enjoying the sun. The client is told that in order to be just as impervious to the rains of life as the ducks are impervious to the rains of the sky, all that he has to do is to set up the suggestion that, from now on, whenever one of those smaller irritations of life comes his way, the image of the ducks will come to mind and immediately, automatically, the petty irritation will simply "run off his back" just like water off the ducks' backs.

The Red Balloon Technique is another wholesale desensitization technique. It was devised by Shelby Walch (1976). The hypnotized client is told that he will see a sturdy container, into which he will place a large portion of his guilt or other unpleasant feelings. The container is slowly filled. Then the client is told to visualize a large red balloon which he slowly inflates with helium. He is told to picture the balloon getting larger and larger as it is inflated. When the balloon is completely inflated, the client is directed to attach the container full of his guilt feelings to the balloon. He is then instructed to hold tightly onto the container and to feel the balloon tugging as it struggles to pull away from him. Next, he is told to loosen his grip on the container and watch the balloon break away and float skyward. Further suggestions are given that as the balloon floats higher and higher it becomes smaller and smaller, until only a small red dot is visible in the sky and then it is completely out of sight.

Visually Hallucinated Symbol As A Deconditioning Method

Moss (1960) reported the use of this technique with a client who sought treatment for a lifelong, intense fear of dogs. The client was given the posthypnotic suggestion that between sessions, whenever she was alone and desired to reestablish her acquaintance with the dog of her early childhood, she could experience a vivid visual hallucination of him. It was emphasized that the dog symbolized her disturbed history, and that this hallucinated relationship provided her with the opportunity to make peace with the past. It was also emphasized that she had complete control of the relationship and could visualize the dog as close as she desired or keep him as distant as her fear dictated.

A Modeling Technique

This fantasy technique may be utilized for any type of disorder. Ludwig, Lyle and Miller (1964) used a modeling technique in the treatment of drug addiction. Subjects were instructed to mentally watch a TV show in which the hero, played by them, was a drug addict who was trying to overcome his addiction. They were instructed to see a situation in which the hero was tempted to take drugs after some type of rejection. Instead, he would overcome the craving and the TV program would show how he achieved it.

The Branding Iron Technique

Ludwig, Lyle and Miller (1964) employed two approaches with an imaginary branding iron in the treatment of drug addiction. In the first approach, patients were told that they were holding a branding iron over the fire, that the iron was becoming red hot and that they would soon be branding their brains with the words *I must never take that first shot of drugs*. They were told to apply the branding iron to their forehead and that these words would be indelibly stamped on their brains forever. They were also told that if they ever experienced a craving for drugs again, these words would blaze in their brains and enhance their willpower to resist drugs.

In the other approach with the imaginary branding iron, patients were told to put their own words on the branding iron and then to brand their brains. Patients chose such phrases as *I will never take that first shot, self-love, stay away from the old environment, drugs and jail are married together, there's no divorce, achieve the goals I'm striving for,* and *get rid of weaknesses.*

INDUCED HALLUCINATIONS OF IMPROVEMENT

Clients with chronic complaints can often be helped by the induction of hallucinations of improvement. In this way, the client can "see" that there is a state of living better than his present state of illness.

The nature of the hallucinations will depend on the patient's symptoms. If, for example, the patient suffers from a skin rash, he can be made to see the condition of his skin improving. With this technique, as with any hallucinatory or scene visualization technique, it is necessary that the client let the therapist know when he experiences the appropriate hallucination. A simple procedure is to tell the client that his right index finger will rise when he can see his present condition (i.e., skin rash) clearly. Then he is told to look at the rash and that as he continues to look at it, it starts to fade. Then he is told that as the rash fades to the point where he can barely see it, his left index finger will rise.

If the client is anxious, it should be suggested that he see himself in a calm and relaxed state. If he suffers from insomnia, he should see himself lying in bed, very calm and comfortable as sleep envelops him.

SENSORY-IMAGERY CONDITIONING

Through the use of scene visualization and sensory imagery, the client learns to control his own feedback systems. Kline (1955) described the use of sensory-imagery conditioning in a person with neurodermatitis of 21 years duration. She felt that her past was so confused and unpleasant that she wished "not to deal with it and to leave it be." Her only request was to help her with her hands, if that was possible.

> Treatment was undertaken on the patient's terms. A light hypnosis was induced rapidly. Further induction succeeded in only slightly deepening the trance state. While in hypnosis the patient was told that her hands would (a) 'start to grow larger and larger until they were very large,' then she was told that they would (b) 'start to become very warm—warmer and warmer and warmer until they were hot,' then (c) 'they would grow very cold—so cold that she would feel them almost freezing,' and then (d) 'they would grow

very large again.' A return to normal size with none of the treatment sensations present was the final step.

In conjunction with these directions, the patient was asked to visualize the hands becoming large, cold, warm and then large again. She reported that she did not think she felt any changes in her hands during the hypnosis but she could visualize these changes in imagery. Posthypnotic directions were given for the sensations described above to manifest themselves, along with the imagery, on each day between treatment sessions. The patient was seen once a week. At no time was any suggestion or direction given as to any improvement in the skin condition. The only activity that was suggested was that of sensory and imagery activity. [p. 186]

After six weeks of sensory-imagery conditioning, the patient's hands had cleared completely.

SYMPTOM SUBSTITUTION

This involves intentional manipulation of symptomatology in those who are, for various reasons, inaccessible to a total therapeutic approach. Symptom substitution should be used to "trade down" to a less handicapping symptom. By trading down, it makes it much easier to give up the symptom. The following types usually respond well to symptom substitution: the poorly motivated client, the "psychotherapy veteran," the client who desperately needs to keep his disability and the geriatric patient.

Kroger (1963) cited the case of an extremely depressed and suicidal 60-year-old male who complained bitterly of a pain in his left foot. He continually "cracked" the bones in his foot to relieve the pain. An orthopedic evaluation was negative. He was given the posthypnotic suggestion to crack the knuckles of his left hand. The pain in his foot cleared up as soon as his attention was shifted to his hand.

Symptom substitution is most suitable for patients who desperately need a neurotic disability in order to face their life situations. No possibility exists for the correction of causative underlying maladjustments. As a therapy, symptom substitution consists of substitution for the existing neurotic disability another one that is comparable in kind, nonincapacitating in character and symptomatically satisfying.

SYMPTOM TRANSFORMATION

Although symptom transformation appears to be similar to symptom substitution, it differs significantly in that there is a utilization of neurotic behavior by a transformation of the personality purposes it serves without an attack upon the symptomatology itself.

When planning to use symptom transformation, the hypnotic operator should teach the client how to control specific ideomotor and ideosensory activities, such as alterations in shape and size of limbs, changes in body temperature and breathing. When the client realizes that he can produce these changes, he is then able to accept the fact that he can remove or develop other somatization reactions by means of self-hypnosis.

Symptom transformation should never be attempted until the client can follow posthypnotic suggestions and manifest posthypnotic amnesia.

Erickson (1954c) described the case of a young man who was unable to urinate unless he did so by applying an eight- or ten-inch wooden or iron pipe to the head of his penis and then urinating through the tube. In hypnosis, he was urged to secure a length of bamboo twelve inches long and to mark it on the outside in quarter inches and to use that in urinating. The client's acceptance of the longer tube constituted an acknowledgement that the therapist could do something about the tube, namely, make it longer. Equally significant was the unrecognized implication that the therapist could make it shorter. Also, the tube was to be bamboo, not wood or iron. Three transformation processes—longer, shorter and material—had been initiated.

The patient was told to hold the bamboo tube with his thumb and forefinger, alternately with the right and left hand as convenient and to flex the other three fingers around the shaft of the penis. He was also told that in a day or two or a week or two he might consider how long the bamboo needed to be and whether or not he could saw off one quarter, one half or even one inch, but that he not feel compelled to do so. He was also told to be certain that he have the three fingers grasping the shaft of the penis so that he could notice better the flow of urine through the bamboo. The session was closed with two final posthypnotic suggestions. One was directed to a total amnesia for the entire hypnotic experience. The other was concerned with the purchasing and preparation of the bamboo with no conscious understanding of the purpose.

About three months later, the patient returned to the therapist and reported that he had been greatly astonished and bewildered to find himself buying the bamboo. He practiced urinating with the bamboo tube for about a week and then reached the conclusion that he could saw off about one half inch and was puzzled when he sawed off a full inch. He wondered when he would saw off some more and suddenly realized that it would be on a Thursday. At that time, he sawed off two inches and several days later another inch. At the end of the month, he had a quarter inch ring of bamboo left. While using it one day, he realized that the flexion of the three fingers around the shaft of the penis gave him a natural tube. He then discarded the remains of the bamboo tube and took great delight in urinating freely and comfortably.

The entire procedure and its outcome demonstrate the ease and effectiveness with which symptomatology can be utilized to secure a transformation of a neurotic problem.

Symptom Amelioration

The technique of symptom amelioration may be of value when there has been a surrender of the personality to an overwhelming symptom-complex formation, making the person inaccessible to intensive therapy.

Erickson (1954c) described how he used symptom amelioration in a case of glove anesthesia extending up to the elbow of the right arm and rapid flexion and extension of that arm. The patient was a 17-year-old mentally retarded male (IQ 65). Efforts made to reduce the frequency of his arm movements (135 times a minute) were unsuccessful. Likewise, any efforts to discuss his problem or to elicit any information failed. It was then that Erickson devised the technique of symptom amelioration: it was suggested that the rate would be increased from 135 to 145 per minute, and that this increased rate would persist until the patient was seen again. At the next session, it was suggested that the arm movement would decrease to the usual 135 until seen again. It was again increased to 145 and again decreased to 135. After several such repetitions, further progress was made by suggesting alternating increments and decrements of 5 and 10 points respectively in the rate of the arm movement. This was continued until a rate of 10 per minute was reached. Then the procedure was reversed to increase the rate to 50 arm movements per minute. Then it was reversed to reduce the rate to 10 per minute. It was then suggested that this rate of 10 per minute would continue for a few days, drop to 5 per minute and then increase to 20 or 30 or more a day. A few days later, the rate shifted from 5 per minute to scattered isolated movements per day, the daily total averaging around 25. Then it was suggested that this count would diminish day by day until it was around 5, and then it would "increase" to as high as 25 times a week. After responding as suggested, the patient was asked to "guess" on what day there would be no uncontrolled movements. He guessed the day when no movements would occur and demonstrated the correctness of his conjecture. The glove anesthesia increased and decreased in direct relation to the arm movement and vanished along with that symptom.

SYMPTOM UTILIZATION

This technique was devised by Milton Erickson (1965). He described the basic premise of symptom utilization:

> The patient's needs as a human personality should be an ever-present question for the therapist to insure recognition at each manifestation. Merely to make a correct diagnosis of the illness and to know the correct method of treatment is not enough. Fully as important is that the patient be receptive of the therapy and cooperative in regard to it. Without the patient's full cooperativeness, therapeutic results are delayed, distorted, limited, or even prevented. [p. 57]

Symptom utilization techniques are particularly suited for stressful situations or for those not amenable to direct hypnotic symptom removal. Symptom utilization consists of encouraging, accepting and redefining behavior in order to control it. It utilizes the patient's own attitudes, feelings and behavior.

Erickson (1959) has developed a number of utilization techniques. The following is an example of Erickson's use of symptom utilization. A male patient in his early thirties entered Dr. Erickson's office and began pacing the floor. He stated that he could not endure relating his problems sitting quietly or lying on a couch and that he had repeatedly been discharged by other psychiatrists because they "accused" him of being uncooperative. He requested hypnotherapy because his anxiety was almost unendurable and increased in intensity in a psychiatrist's office, making it necessary for him to constantly pace the floor.

The therapist asked to participate in his pacing by the measure of directing it in part. To this the client agreed. Then he was asked to pace back and forth, to turn to the right, to turn to the left, to walk away from the chair, and to walk toward it. At first, these instructions were given in a tempo matching the client's step. Gradually, the tempo of the suggestions was slowed and the wording was changed: "Now turn to the right away from the chair in which you can sit; turn left toward the chair in which you can sit; walk away from the chair in which you can sit." The tempo was then slowed more and the wording was again changed to include the phrase: "the chair which you will soon approach as if to seat yourself comfortably," which in turn was altered to "the chair in which you will shortly find yourself sitting comfortably." In this way, the client's pacing became progressively slower and more dependent upon the therapist's instructions until direct suggestions could be given that he seat himself in the chair and go deeper into hypnosis as he related his history.

The primary value of symptom utilization lies in its effective demonstration to the client that he is completely acceptable and that the therapist can deal effectively with him regardless of his behavior.

Methods for the use of symptom substitution, symptom transformation, symptom amelioration, and symptom utilization in the management of obesity are provided by Kroger (1970). In symptom substitution, one can "trade down" to other eating behaviors such as chewing gum or becoming interested in the taste of dietetic foods. In symptom transformation, overeating can be transferred by appropriate posthypnotic suggestions to other behaviors such as physical exercise, interest in community affairs, etc. In symptom amelioration, the overeating is reduced. First, it is increased by posthypnotic suggestion on the supposition that if it can be increased voluntarily, it can also be decreased voluntarily. Symptom utilization in the management of obesity consists of encouraging, accepting and redefining cooperative activity of an aversive nature toward faulty eating patterns.

A number of other techniques can be adapted to direct hypnotherapy. The field is as broad as the therapist's imagination.

Chapter 13.

Hypnoidal Hypnoanalysis

In hypnoidal hypnoanalysis, the client is in a hypnoidal state or only in a light stage of hypnosis. Hypnoidal hypnoanalysis is indicated for those individuals who are in need of a hypnoanalytic treatment approach, but who are either incapable of reaching the depth of hypnosis required for reconstructive hypnoanalysis or for whom a formal hypnotic induction procedure is contraindicated. One of the major advantages of the hypnoidal state is that it can be induced without reference to hypnosis.

Hypnoidal hypnoanalysis is specifically indicated for schizoid individuals, prepsychotics, individuals who have formed strong misconceptions about hypnosis and those incapable of achieving a deep state of hypnosis whose symptoms are the manifestations of active psychological conflict.

The procedures for inducing the hypnoidal state and for arousing the client from the hypnoidal state have already been presented in the chapter on hypnoidal therapy and will not be repeated at this time.

Hypnoidal hypnoanalysis may be conducted in a question-and-answer fashion. Other techniques that may be employed in hypnoidal hypnoanalysis are hypnotic dreaming, directed association, guided fantasy techniques, hypnogogic reveries, and hypnointrospection. All of these techniques are designed to get at repressed material, but they require only a very light stage of hypnosis. With highly motivated

101

clients, a hypnoanalysis may be conducted in a light stage of hypnosis when the techniques of hypnoidal hypnoanalysis are employed.

Hypnotic Dreaming

It should be suggested to the client that he have a dream while in the hypnoidal state during the session. This procedure involves hypnotic suggestion as opposed to posthypnotic suggestion.

When giving suggestions for dreaming in the hypnoidal state, the therapist should state the particular problem, for the client may be experiencing active fantasy, and therefore might be misled into dreaming of some other subject. Also, if the suggestion to dream is left completely open, the client may dream of some inconsequential subject as a defense. After stating the particular problem, the therapist should give the following instructions to the client in the hypnoidal state: "You are deeply relaxed . . . calm and relaxed. I will leave you for ten minutes while you dream. You will dream a dream which will answer the problem. You are dreaming now." At the conclusion of the ten-minute period, the therapist should ask the client to relate his dream while he remains in the hypnoidal state.

In addition to artificially inducing dreams while the client is in the hypnoidal state, dreams may be posthypnotically suggested to appear later during nocturnal sleep, or they may be posthypnotically suggested to appear during a natural sleep state induced by suggestion in the hypnoanalytic session. Both types of posthypnotically suggested dreaming require a somnambulistic stage of hypnosis and are utilized during reconstructive hypnoanalysis.

Directed Association

In hypnosis, associations are often directed by the therapist so that they are less free. For example, the client in the hypnoidal state may be told that he will see an image applicable to the situation immediately after the therapist has counted to five. Or the client may be instructed to visualize a chalkboard in front of him and told that he will see words appear on the chalkboard. If resistance is still encountered, it can be suggested that single letters will appear in a scrambled fashion but will make up a word when unscrambled. The client might then name the letters, whereupon the therapist states that he is going to count to five and upon the count of five the letters will move into their proper order to make a meaningful word.

An excellent example of directed association is the letter-association technique developed by Dr. Edward Dengrove (1962). The client is asked to close his eyes and to relax as much as possible. He is then asked to think of a particular symptom, to relate it to the last situation in which it was felt, and to attempt to relive to whatever extent possible the feeling of the complaint.

Then he is asked to give the very first letter that comes to mind. The letter is noted and the client is then asked to give the next letter that comes to mind. A total of five letters of the alphabet are given. Then the letters are listed vertically in order. The client is then requested to give the first word that comes to mind that begins with each of the letters previously chosen.

After the five words have been noted separately, the usual word association technique is used. The words usually form a battery of information related to the original difficulty.

Dengrove gives the example of this technique with a 37-year-old housewife who presented complaints of "ungodly thoughts going through my head. I sit and cry and cry and cry, and I don't know why." Asked to give five letters, she produced the following and their subsequent associations:

F   Free—Boat won't let me be free financially.
G   Good—It's good for my husband. He enjoys it.
P   Poor—It's making us broke.
B   Boat—The same thing.
B   Bob—My husband.

This led to the precipitating event of her depressed state, which was the purchase of a boat by her husband with the consequent strain upon their finances. Further exploration led to her conflicts with him and the use of the boat purchase as the excuse for expressing her antagonism toward him.

GUIDED FANTASY TECHNIQUES

These techniques are extremely suitable for use in hypnoidal hypnoanalysis. The principal developers of these techniques have been Carl Happich, Robert Desoille and Hanscarl Leuner.

Happich developed his techniques of guided fantasy, which he called symbolic consciousness, from his literary and practical knowledge of Oriental techniques. He combined Oriental wisdom with the experience of modern depth psychology. Happich set forth his fundamental principles in two small books, published in 1932 and 1939, which unfortunately have never been translated from German into English. The exposition presented here of Happich's techniques is based upon Wolfgang Kretschmer's discussion in his paper on meditative techniques in psychotherapy (1969). Kretschmer stated:

> Happich took the level of consciousness he called "Symbolic consciousness," which seems to lie between consciousness and unconsciousness, as the point of departure for all creative production and, therefore, also for the healing process. On this level the "collective unconscious" can express itself through symbolism. [p. 220]

Happich encouraged, both before and during the scenes, an increasing passivity of respiration. For most individuals, this can be achieved only through progressive breathing exercises.

With the client in a hypnoidal state with eyes closed, it is suggested that he visualize himself in a series of scenes. The therapist suggests scenes that have symbolic and therapeutic import and are related to basic aspects of intrapsychic and interpersonal functioning. The following scenes are most often used: (1) a meadow; (2) climbing a mountain; (3) visiting a chapel; (4) visiting a house; (5) following the course of a stream, and (6) watching the eruption of a volcano. Any scene that spontaneously suggests itself to the client is also appropriate.

The client should be fully prepared for the experience of fantasy, including an explanation of the mechanics of the process. Kelly (1972) mentioned four major points which should be adhered to in the preparation of the client for guided fantasy. First, the client should be introduced to the technique along the following lines: "This is a fantasy approach that may give us some new insights into your thoughts and feelings. It is nothing mysterious."

Second, the client should understand his functioning in the technique. The therapist might say, "First I'll give you a scene to deal with. The important thing is to let your imagination go where it wants to as it develops the experience. Don't try to make it go where you think it ought to. Try to visualize and fully experience the scene. I may make suggestions from time to time, but you are free to reject them."

Third, the client should be prepared to experience feelings. He may be told: "Be sure to let yourself really experience the feelings you have. Don't be surprised if you feel intense emotions. Let your-self really feel them."

Fourth, the client's freedom, autonomy, and control should be emphasized. In order to emphasize these characteristics in the client, the therapist may say, "Keep in mind that you are in full control of the situation. You can stop the fantasy anytime you want. You will experience emotions only because you are letting yourself experi-ence them."

After visualizing himself in each scene, the client is then asked to describe it in detail and to relate the events that follow. What-ever is unresolved at a subconscious level of awareness will manifest itself via symbolic visual forms and proceed to resolve itself at the symbolic level.

In his fantasy, the client may move in various directions in psy-chological space and thus confront, intrapsychically, the hidden depths and highest potentialities of his intra-psychic functioning.

Desoille (1965) stated that in order to reeducate emotional re-sponses, the first prerequisite is to evoke the client's habitual re-sponses and thereby to define the client's potentialities in the emotional domain. Verbalization in the normal waking state is not a favorable condition for the free expression of feelings and emo-tions. This is best accomplished in the hypnoidal state, as in symbolic consciousness.

One who is familiar with dream symbolism—and these tech-niques demand of the therapist ample experience in and understand-ing of dream interpretation—will recognize that these scenes are highly symbolic.

The meadow represents the blossoming of life that the client seeks. It also represents the world and the creative power of the child. Every healthy individual has in his psychic depths something cor-responding to the meadow. He retains within himself an active and creative child. When an individual is psychically ill, the child loses its positive and creative power. Thus, the psychically ill find it impossible to visualize a fresh meadow and cannot find one. As the client improves psychically, the meadow improves. The grass be-comes green and the flowers and trees bloom.

Climbing the mountain symbolizes a movement during which the client demonstrates his capacity to develop toward the goal of psychic freedom. Psychically disturbed individuals will be confronted by many obstacles in their climb to the top. As the client improves, he is progressively able to overcome the obstacles and climb to the top, usually describing feelings that are extremely elevating.

In the chapel scene, the client is led into the innermost rooms of his psyche, where he faces the question of how he relates to the possibilities of psychic transformation. When the individual is able to comprehend the symbolic significance of the chapel, he can use it to uncover and face in himself the central problems of life.

The house may stand for the parents' home, the client's soul or his past. It usually symbolizes the self: the various rooms will represent the various compartments of self. Exploring the attic and cellar as well as opening locked closets can help the client confront symbolically various aspects of his hidden and unintegrated self. This is also true for exploring the depths of an ocean, a cave or a forest.

In following the course of a stream, going upstream may be similar to climbing a mountain with many obstacles, or the stream may exert a soothing or stimulating influence: the client may take a cleansing bath (i.e., of his psychic tensions).

Watching the eruption of a volcano presents the chance for hostile, destructive discharges, that later on become reconstructive.

There are five basic principles of symbolic consciousness: (1) symbol confrontation; (2) the principle of feeding; (3) the principle of reconciliation; (4) the principle of the magic fluids, and (5) the principle of exhausting and killing.

Symbol confrontation is a way of dealing with the symbolic figures that emerge from the forest, cave or ocean. It is a very strong, active technique that requires a therapist who is able to tolerate strong emotional outbursts from his clients. When confronted by a frightful creature, the client is told to stare into the eyes of the creature and at the same time to describe it in detail. There is a twofold purpose of persistent staring into the eyes of the creature: first, to discover the meaning that the creature's existence conveys, and second, to banish the creature from one's fantasies. During this confrontation, the therapist actively supports the client. By demanding a detailed and accurate description of the frightening image, he forces the client to replace his archaic anxiety with an analytical attitude, which is effective for reality testing. The end result of the successful symbol confrontation is a strengthening of the ego.

The principle of "feeding" is a more passive way of subduing the threat, but is active enough to help those clients who feel too vulnerable for symbol confrontation. It is a good way for a client to deal with symbolic figures perceived as being aggressive or dangerous. When the client is faced with an angry or potentially dangerous symbolic figure, it is suggested that he feed the creature. It is the task of the client to feed the creature as much as possible so that it gets drowsy and loses its aggressiveness.

The purpose of the principle of reconciliation is to make friends with hostile symbolic figures by petting or stroking them and showing tenderness toward them in various ways.

The feared symbolic figure usually represents some part of the client himself, usually a derivative of a parent introject. Making friends with the symbolic figure means assimilating this introject, which has been rejected and projected onto the symbolic figure.

Following the course of a stream symbolizes the flow of psychic energy. With the psychically ill client, the stream never flows down to the ocean without some kind of obstruction. The path back to the spring may be defined as a regression back to the source of psychic energy. The water pouring forth from the spring refreshes the weary traveler, and he finds strength from drinking the imaginary water. Besides spring water, there are other magic fluids, such as cow's milk and mother's milk.

The principle of exhausting and killing is usually successful in handling acute conflicts at the time of therapy. Hanscarl Leuner (1966) showed how this technique was used with a 34-year-old woman suffering from hypochondria, following a car accident which made her feel that she would soon die. During her visualization, she saw a skeleton emerge out of the trunk of the tree against which her car had crashed. This symbol of death came forth into the daydream and threatened the client, who, at the therapist's urging, pursued it and forced it to run into the countryside. When it wanted to sit down for a rest, it was pushed on. At last the skeleton arrived at a river bank and fell into the river. The water dissolved its bones. The client improved dramatically after this session.

Hammer (1967) reported the extension of guided fantasy to include symbolic role playing of every element in the fantasy. With this technique, the client is asked to imagine that he is the person, animal, creature or natural setting (stream, meadow, mountain, etc.) he has visualized and to enact the scene from that point of view. According to Hammer, the technique of symbolic role playing is useful for reintegrating projected material, for working through anxiety-arousing images, for improving interpersonal relationships and for gaining insight into the meaning of the symbolic representations.

Hypnagogic Reverie

Kubie (1943) has shown that a state of hypnagogic reverie can bring about easier access to subconscious material.

The hypnagogic reverie is a dream without distortion. Through the induction of states of hypnagogic reverie, significant information about the past can be made readily accessible, without the need for interpretations, which are requisite in the translation of dreams.

A simple physiological method for the induction of hypnagogic reveries has been described by Kubie (1943). In this method, the subject's own breath sounds are picked up by a microphone placed against the neck; they are amplified and brought back to the subject through earphones. In most individuals, the sound and rhythm of their own breathing, used as a fixating stimulus, has a powerful hypnagogic influence.

In a paper on the use of hypnagogic reveries in the recovery of repressed amnesic data, Kubie stated:

> The hypnagogic reverie might be called a dream without distortion. Its immediate instigator is the day's "unfinished business," but like the dream it derives from more remote "unfinished business" of an entire lifetime as well. The hypnagogic reverie differs from a dream in the fact that there is less elision of the remote and recent past, and far less use of symbolic representation. This would seem to be due to two facts: in the first place, since the reverie does not attempt to say as much as a dream, it does not need to depend upon condensed hieroglyphics to express multiple meanings. In the second place, when the hypnagogic reverie is artificially induced for therapeutic purposes, guilt and anxiety seem to play a less active role than in a dream, with the result that the content of the reverie can come through with less disguise. Whatever the

explanation, the consequence is that through the induction of states of hypnagogic reverie, significant information about the past can be made readily and directly accessible, without depending upon the interpretations which are requisite in the translation of dreams. [1943, p. 172]

Hypnagogic reverie sessions commence by asking the client to remain silent, listening to his own amplified breath sounds. He is then asked to count his breath sounds silently to himself: "one, two, one, two" or "in and out, in and out." After about ten minutes, the client is asked what has been going on. After he relates his feelings and thoughts he is again asked to be silent, to listen to his breathing as before, and to use his own final statement as the starting point for his thoughts. He is told that the therapist might break in on his silence at any time to ask him what is going on, but that if there is anything that he wants to communicate, he should signal.

This technique is suitable either for clients who are unable to reach a somnambulistic depth or in whom repressed material has remained inaccessible through other hypnoanalytic techniques.

HYPNOINTROSPECTION

Hypnointrospection is a neuromuscular hypnoanalytic technique developed by Dr. Seymour Halpern (1967). When using the hypno-introspective approach, the client assumes a supine posture on the couch with legs extended, arms close to the body, fingers together and palms down, the neck comfortably extended, the tongue brought to the floor of the mouth, the eyes closed and shoes removed. After the hypnointrospective posture has been attained, the client is instructed to maintain it. The client is then asked to direct his attention to the body and objectify all events by reporting them according to category, i.e., sensations, affects, thoughts and images. When unpleasant or painful events are experienced, the client is encouraged to receive them fully. If the client complains of feelings of emptiness, he is told to experience them fully. This leads to discernible changes in bodily expression. The feeling of emptiness is only one of the many expressions of anxiety that tend to disrupt hypnointrospection. When this happens, it is effective to have the client focus his attention on the stomach or mouth and throat. Concentrating on the stomach or mouth reduces visceral tensions quickly and results in the abatement of anxiety.

Hypnointrospection views conflicts as postural, and therefore calls attention to an arching back or a clenched fist, which aids the client in maintaining the associative process.

By concentrating on bodily feelings and working from the gut outward, i.e., from the involuntary to the voluntary muscles, the client is helped in the stabilization and extension of self-control.

The aim of hypnointrospection is to facilitate and maintain the associative process with a minimal disruption of ego control. Hypnointrospection is organized around a twofold system of frustration: (1) the inner dialogue during which the client learns to come to terms with his body, and (2) the outer dialogue in which he learns to come to terms with society and to expand the rational basis of his experience. Through a systematic and intensive relationship, the therapist seeks and hopes to foster optimal self-control on the part of the client. "In the course of the outer dialogue," stated Halpern, "the patient is brought to the realization that much of his illness constitutes a rejection of his body—a rejection based on fear and ignorance. He is encouraged to face these fears, to overcome this ignorance and to appreciate the healing potentialities of his body." [1967, p. 82]

Halpern found corroboration for an observation that contributed largely to the development of hypnointrospection. This observation was that talking about feelings, although facilitating cognitive control over behavior, diminishes affective intensity by distracting from the immediacy of the experience. Thus, the traditional technique of free association in its orthodox application is intrinsically self-restricting.

Reports of visual imagery and their subsequent analysis are standard aspects of the hypnointrospective technique. Halpern has reported great individual variation, in form and in content, of the visual imagery. Many clients report body image perceptions only. Some report darkness with flashes of color.

The qualified use of hypnointrospection offers the client an unprecedented degree of self-control and a significant mitigation of unanticipated anxiety reactions. While learning hypnointrospection, the client develops an orientation in the art of becoming his own authority. In being free to feel, he is concurrently free to think. The client is assisted by the therapist in acquiring self-discipline, which can lead him to greater awareness. He learns to introspect and to consider his experiences in terms of information.

In his discussion of the innovative aspects of hypnointrospection, Halpern (1967) stated:

> In seeking to isolate the significant elements in our procedure, it became evident that the alteration of sensory-tonic relations and the identification of the affective elements during the hypnointrospective state were crucial. Since the identification of affect long has been established as a prepotent factor in therapy, the alteration of sensory-tonic states through voluntary inhibition of movement was identified as the essential innovation. [141-42]

The main potential danger in hypnoidal hypnoanalysis is that hypnosis is so light that subconscious material may rise to the threshold of conscious awareness, causing the client to awaken abruptly. This may precipitate an acute anxiety reaction. In the event that this happens, the therapist should immediately rehypnotize the client using an authoritarian approach and give suggestions of calmness and relaxation. In order for hypnoidal hypnoanalysis to be successful, the client must be well motivated and have sufficient understanding of the psychodynamic processes involved so that he can cooperate intelligently and make a conscious effort to maintain the hypnoidal state. This method should be used only with individuals who have a sufficient amount of ego strength, because posthypnotic amnesia cannot be induced in such a light trance.

Chapter 14.

Reconstructive Hypnoanalysis

Reconstructive hypnoanalysis aims at a reconstructive change in personality. It aims not only at restoration of the individual to a level of effective life functioning, but it strives also to bring about a maturation of emotional development with the creation of new adaptive potentialities. Insight into subconscious conflicts with efforts to achieve extensive alterations of the character structure is the primary goal.

Reconstructive hypnoanalysis is applicable in every instance where a dynamic and extensive investigation of the personality is wanted. Also, the client must be highly motivated for this type of treatment and must have a sufficient amount of ego strength.

The hypnoanalytic techniques utilized depend to a large extent on the client's development as a hypnotic subject, and on the type of disorder and its severity. A brief description will be given of the following hypnoanalytic techniques: age regression, the hypnoanalytic utilization of dreams, techniques of graphic expresssion, techniques of plastic expression, hallucinatory techniques, most-or-least method, hypnotic intensification of emotion, production of experimental conflict, hypnotic play therapy, the affect-bridge technique, narcohypnoanalysis, projective hypnoanalysis, and the hypnotic manipulation of ego cathexis.

AGE REGRESSION

Age regression ranks as one of the most important methods in hypnoanalysis. There are two types of age regression: the memory type and the revivification type. In the memory type of age regression, the client is brought back to some earlier period of his life. The client uses the past tense and recalls incidents from that particular time of his life. In revivification, the client returns to a former period of his life and relives his past experiences. Age regression is beneficial as a means of obtaining a catharsis for emotional trauma and as a means of uncovering repressed memories associated with a traumatic event. When hunting for the trauma by this technique, LeCron and Bordeaux (1947) suggested that the client be regressed to a period prior to the appearance of his symptoms and then carried forward again in time until the cause appears. After this is revealed, the client is kept regressed while conflicts are probed. Positive suggestions should be given to counteract any negative suggestions that the client may have accepted at the period of life to which he has regressed, as a result of the emotional trauma.

The Hypnoanalytic Utilization of Dreams

The study of dreams is an important part of hypnoanalysis. Dreams may be artificially induced during hypnosis; they may be posthypnotically suggested to appear later during nocturnal sleep; or they may be posthypnotically suggested to appear during a natural sleep state induced by suggestion in the hypnoanalytic session. Hartman (1967) has reported the following procedure. To accustom a client to the production of dreams, first a posthypnotic suggestion is given him to the effect that in his sleep the night before the next hypnoanalytic session, he will have a dream that will reveal an important aspect of his problem, and that he will remember the dream and report it at the next session. If this suggestion is followed, it is repeated, and the client is given a specific topic to dream about. After the client has learned to dream in this fashion, the next step is to induce sleep by suggestion. The client is put into a somnambulistic state and then given sleep suggestions to occur after he is aroused from the hypnotic state. He is told that after he is aroused from the hypnotic state, when the word *sleep* is said he will fall into a natural sleep and will have a dream on a specific topic. Wolberg (1945) claimed that the client's spontaneous dreams occurring immediately after initiation of treatment often will contain the crux of the whole problem—the central conflict and the basis of the neurosis. Induced dreams are most suitable for cases in which age regression and abreaction cannot be induced.

TECHNIQUES OF GRAPHIC EXPRESSION

There are a number of techniques of graphic expression. Our discussion will include the following: automatic writing, writing in trance and post-hypnotic writing, and hypnography. These techniques are most suitable for clients who have difficulty verbalizing in hypnoanalysis or who are not adept at the hallucinatory techniques.

Automatic Writing This technique is of value when a situation arises in analysis which can be solved by the expression of a single word or phrase. The hypnotized client is told that the arm and hand with which he writes will feel as if they are no longer a part of him. Then a pencil is placed in his hand and he is told that his hand will begin to move as if it were controlled by some outside force. Generally the first few attempts produce a jumble of lines and symbols, gradually increasing in freedom of expression as the motor activity becomes better established. The subconscious mind will often use various devices to make it difficult for the therapist to decipher the records. It is best, therefore, to have the client explain the meaning of his automatic writing while still in hypnosis. A few of the subconscious disguises which have been uncovered in automatic writing are: writing upside down, writing words backwards, and repetition of one letter or syllable.

After automatic writing is well developed, it often relates whole repressed episodes of early childhood in a coherent fashion. Reports have been made of clear impressions from the first year of life, which have been confirmed by family members. At times, especially when the meaning is disguised even to the hypnotized person, it is beneficial to have him associate to the material. The client may then be asked whether he wants to remember the meaning of the automatic writing when he is awakened from hypnosis. The subconscious mind is a good judge of the strength of the ego and its ability to cope with the uncovering of material from the subconscious level of awareness. This technique was explained in detail by Muhl (1965).

Writing in Trance and Posthypnotic Writing These methods are effective methods of clarification of material when meaningful material has been produced, but they leave both the client and therapist uncertain about its relationship to the present. Stolzheise (1961) gave the following procedure to use when utilizing these methods.

> If the patient is in deep trance, he may be instructed to open his eyes, move to the writing desk, and write what the subconscious wants him to understand clearly in the waking state. He is to continue to write until the subconscious permits him to lay down his pen, and then he is to awaken with full clarity. Sometimes a dissertation is written, or the production may be only a repetition of a word or words. If the patient is in a medium trance or lighter, he can be instructed for posthypnotic writing, using approximately the same instructions. There should be enough repetition and emphasis to insure a prompt attempt to write when the patient is awakened. If it is convenient, the patient can be left to do the writing and then turn it in to the secretary, as a timesaving mechanism. The writing is a powerful emphasis to the patient of his own part in the therapy and causes him to be more thoughtfully active at home on his own. [258-59]

Hypnography   Developed by Meares (1957), this graphic technique of hypnoanalysis involves the hypnotized person projecting psychic material in black-and-white painting. The main indication for hypnography is the inability of the client to talk freely in verbal hypnoanalysis. When the client expresses his conflicts in painting, verbal expression becomes much easier. Meares (1960) stated that hypnography should also be considered in cases in which the client cannot adjust to a present-day reality conflict. By confronting the problem when he expresses it in hypnotic painting, the client develops a greater tolerance of the conflict. The object is to get him to paint something that represents traumatic material, either repressed material or that of which he is aware but unable to express verbally. The main value of hypnography is in having the client associate to his paintings while still in hypnosis.

TECHNIQUES OF PLASTIC EXPRESSION

These techniques are used for the same reasons for which the techniques of graphic expression are used, with the exception that the techniques of plastic expression more often elicit spontaneous age regression with abreaction than do the graphic techniques. This is most likely due to the primitive nature of the plastic techniques; it would be explained by the atavistic theory of hypnosis of Meares

(1960). The techniques of plastic expression include hypnoplasty (Meares, 1960), and sensory hypnoplasty (Raginsky, 1961).

Hypnoplasty This is an excellent approach for the resistant client. It is a technique in hypnoanalysis in which the hypnotized person uses clay to model whatever he desires. Then he is asked to associate to the clay model. In this way, the meaning and nature of the conflict that caused the client to make a particular model are revealed. Hypnoplasty is of particular benefit for clients who do not talk readily when in hypnosis. The expression of a conflict in plastic form is usually accompanied by the appropriate emotion, thereby bringing the client to express himself in words.

Sensory hypnoplasty In this hypnoanalytic technique, the hypnotized person models clay, to which various sensory stimuli have been added to stimulate basic primitive memories, associations, sensations and conflicts. Sensory hypnoplasty appears to facilitate regression to the oral and anal stages of development much more rapidly than any other method. This type of regression is not altogether fortuitous, since nonverbal suggestions are created by the color, texture, form, and odor of the clay which is presented to the client when this type of regression is indicated in treatment. The degree of regression as well as its direction can be manipulated easily by changing the type of clay. In this way, one can guide the progress of therapy very subtly into practically any direction or channel the therapist believes is indicated. It happens only occasionally that the client will regress to these early stages automatically without regard to the type of clay he has in his hands. In sensory hypnoplasty, the multiple sensations are increased very markedly by changing the texture of the clay, its temperature, color, smell, and consistency. The addition of sensory stimuli to the clay enhances the dynamic quality of hypnoplasty in a remarkable way. By manipulating the temperature, texture, consistency, color and smell of the clay, one can bring out conflicts dealing with phobias, personal and interpersonal relationships, etc.

HALLUCINATORY TECHNIQUES

Induced hallucinations can be of tremendous benefit in hypnoanalysis. The basic principle is that the client is brought to hallucinate, but the nature of the hallucination is not suggested. The content is determined by the underlying conflicts which are pressing for expression in the client's own subconscious. There are a number of hallucinatory techniques, but our discussion will be confined to the following: crystal and mirror gazing, the motion picture technique, the house technique, the hallucinated unconscious body image, and hallucinated sensory hypnoplasty.

Crystal and Mirror Gazing These are excellent methods of recovering forgotten memories and are of particular value with clients who have brought up repressed incidents through hypnotically induced dreams and automatic writing, but are unable to recall the incidents as real experiences or to accept them as factual. By gazing into a crystal or a mirror, the client is often able to reconstruct events in his past life. A glass of water will serve as an adequate substitute for a crystal. If a mirror is used it should be placed so that it reflects the ceiling. Wolberg (1945) gave the following instructions to his patients: "You will now be able to open your eyes, even though you are deeply asleep. You will not awaken until I give you the command to do so. On the table in front of you, you will see a mirror. Look into the mirror and you will see things before you. Describe to me what you see." [p. 214] Violent emotional reactions may be elicited by this method.

Motion Picture Technique The hypnotized client is told to visualize a movie screen. Gindes (1953), when using this technique, gave the following instructions: "Soon I shall ask you to open your eyes. When you do, you will find that you are in a motion picture theatre. Ahead of you is the screen. On the screen you will see a movie. This motion picture is the story of your life. You will notice that all of the important details of your life have been successively woven into the story that you see before you on the screen. I want you to tell me about them, for I am unable to see the screen. Now I am going to ask you to open your eyes, and just ahead of you, you will see the screen." [p. 228-29] The client opens his eyes and begins to recount everything that he sees on his screen. He gives a vivid account of forgotten experiences. As he visualizes and recounts the incidents, which before were too painful for him to retain at the conscious level of awareness, the client enters suitable abreaction. The client can be led to look at the screen to view the traumatic incident again and again, until he becomes desensitized to it.

In discussing his use of the motion picture technique, Gindes stated: "I have used this method more frequently than any other, having found it to be very much the most satisfactory method of catharsis. The patient, in relating what he sees on the screen, becomes so objective about it that he makes very little attempt to repress either what he sees or his emotions concerning it." [1953, p. 231]

House Technique   The client is led to hallucinate that he is going into a house and is brought to describe what he sees. He will almost always hallucinate the house of his childhood or a house that holds some traumatic memory for him. This is a very effective technique for the uncovering of significant material. It is less structured than the motion picture technique and, therefore, there is less of a tendency for the client to use the setting as a defense. Meares (1960) gave the following instructions: "You are going along the street. You come to the house. You come to the house. It is just as it used to be. You see it as clear as anything. You go to the door. You open the door, and you go in. It is all there. You see it. You see it all. What's happening? Tell me what's happening." [p. 402] This technique can be used as background before proceeding to regression and abreaction.

Hallucinated Unconscious Body Image Technique   This technique was developed by Freytag (1961, 1965). It is suggested to the hypnotized person that he hallucinate a full-length mirror and see his reflection in the mirror. He is then asked to describe what he sees. It is explained that what he sees is a reflection of the external appearance of his spatial body image: he is seeing his body image as it exists in space. Then follows the comment that this body image, which he sees in the mirror, doesn't tell him what he is feeling or experiencing in his subconscious mind. He is then told that each and every one of us has a picture or an image of himself in his subconscious mind, which we will call the unconscious body image. This unconscious body image, however, may differ from the external appearance of the body image as seen in the mirror because the subconscious mind expresses itself in a symbolic fashion. As treatment progresses, the client may be asked to hallucinate an unconscious body image with special reference to a particular area of conflict or a particular complaint. It is frequently important to establish a particular frame of reference. Since the unconscious body images change in response to changes in percepts, the client is able to objectively perceive therapeutic progress in the expressive modifications of his unconscious body image.

The most important factor entering into the development of hallucinated sensory hypnoplasty (Sacerdote & Sacerdote, 1969) was the strong belief that hallucinated experiences involving the various senses may be more effective in directing clients towards deep levels of hypnosis than the real objects, colors or sounds. Sacerdote has found that the observing ego's concern with the possibility of dirtying and damaging the environment is absent in the case of hallucinated sensory hypnoplasty, thus permitting the client to let himself go much more freely. Also, with the disappearance of limitations of time and space, the client can combine, or variously alternate, materials of different size, weight, color, smell, consistency and taste in a practically limitless fashion.

Most-or-Least Method

Some of the questions that may be used to uncover repressed traumatic events are: "About what are you most fearful in your life?" "About what are you most angry in your life?" "What was the guiltiest feeling in your life?" and "What was the most frustrating situation when you were very little?"

Hypnotic Intensification of Emotion

The hypnotic intensification of emotion is an effective technique for clients characterized by what Fenichel (1945) referred to as "feeling phobia." Some clients with a feeling phobia blot out awareness of emotion or of events. In others, emotions may be aroused but not spontaneously felt. If, during treatment, recollection occurs without emotional effect, the hypnotic intensification and recognition of the underlying emotion may be extremely effective. Rosen (1953) stated that in his experience, if the emotion of the moment was hypnotically intensified, sexual fantasies, naked anxiety or pronounced rage reactions came to the surface, frequently to the point of being acted out. When using this technique, Rosen gave the hypnotized person the following instructions: "Whatever your underlying emotion at present, you'll gradually feel it grow stronger, stronger and stronger still, stronger than you've ever felt it before in your life, until it's as strong as you're able to bear it, until you feel it as deeply as it's possible for you to feel any emotion." [p 258] In view of the potential dangers involved, this technique should only be utilized by experienced therapists who have had considerable experience with the other hypnoanalytic techniques.

PRODUCTION OF EXPERIMENTAL CONFLICT

A similar caution as was stated for the intensification of emotion is in order for the production of experimental conflict. Both of these techniques are highly dynamic and potentially dangerous. The production of an experimental conflict, an artificial situation which resembles the client's conflict situation, may give the client sufficient insight as to how and why he reacts to his own conflict. The hypnotized client is told that he is in a situation resembling his area of conflict. He is led to experience the appropriate emotion, and he reacts to it in his own particular neurotic manner. The client is instructed to remember the experiences and feelings that he had while in hypnosis so that he will gain insight into his conflict situation.

HYPNOTIC PLAY THERAPY

This is an excellent technique for the expression of unconscious aggression, for the acting out of jealousies in relation to a parent or sibling, and for the exploration of sexual and excretory fantasies. A deep state of hypnosis is necessary so that the client can open his eyes while remaining in deep hypnosis and manipulate the materials. Hypnotic play therapy may be utilized both at adult and regressed age levels.

THE AFFECT BRIDGE TECHNIQUE

The affect bridge is a hypnoanalytic technique developed by Dr. John Watkins (1971). It can often facilitate the process of association, helping the client to move from present transferred experiences to their earlier origins. When using the affect bridge, the current affect is vivified and all other aspects of the present experience hypnotically ablated. The client is then asked to return to some earlier experience during which the affect was felt and to relive the associated event.

The affect bridge emphasizes the utilization of common elements between present and past experiences that are affective in nature.

The client is encouraged to allow his associations to move along chains of affect, instead of chains of ideas as is usual in psychoanalytic association.

NARCOHYPNOANALYSIS

Narcohypnoanalysis is a combination of narcoanalysis and hypnoanalysis. Narcohypnoanalysis is of value if a patient needs an excuse to let himself talk more freely. Meares (1960) felt that narcohypnoanalysis had a place in the education of the medical hypnoanalyst. According to Meares, it provides a useful training medium for the young doctor who is not too sure of himself yet in dealing with the hypnotized patient.

PROJECTIVE HYPNOANALYSIS

This hypnoanalytic technique utilizes the combined tactics of the three basic approaches to the understanding of unconscious conflicts —psychoanalysis, hypnosis, and projective techniques. It makes use of free association, dream analysis, and transference reactions as they are projected onto relatively unstructured situations in hypnosis. The best subjects for this approach are those with a vivid fantasy life. In projective hypnoanalysis, there is often active intervention by the therapist to suggest a fantasy on any topic desired. The client may choose his own symbols, or he may be given a set of symbols to work with, such as the pictures from the Thematic Apperception Test (TAT—a projective technique consisting of a series of loosely structured pictures, to which the client is encouraged to make up a story about what he sees) or the Rorschach Test (a series of ten ink blots).

Projective tests such as the TAT, Rorschach Test or a word association test may be administered to the hypnotic subject in order to bring underlying drives and ego defenses into sharper focus. It has been found that projective testing in hypnosis offers a more complete evaluation of personality changes during hypnoanalytic treatment. There is an increased perceptiveness for subconscious stimuli in hypnosis, and the test material elicited during hypnosis has been found to be much more revealing of subconscious conflicts than test material elicited in the normal waking state.

Fantasy and dream symbols may be tested by progressive substitution. When a "stranger" appears in a dream or fantasy, the client is asked to put a mask on the stranger of his father's face, mother's face, therapist's face, etc., and see which one fits. A number of other treatment methods are employed with projective hypnoanalysis. For a more detailed account of this technique, refer to Watkins (1965) and Schneck (1965).

THE HYPNOTIC MANIPULATION OF EGO CATHEXIS

This hypnoanalytic technique was developed by Dr. John Watkins (1963 and 1967). The hypnoanalytic relationship is defined by Watkins (1963) as a "co-existential state in which the transactions of communication and encounter are facilitated by the hypnotic manipulation of ego cathexis." [p. 11] "If we are able," Watkins continues, "through hypnotic techniques to invest or withdraw ego cathexis from various mental or bodily contents, then we have a useful tool for moving toward the existential goals of therapy, namely, to live more intensely, to feel more meaningfully, to increasingly 'be' in the Umwelt, the Mitwelt and the Eigenwelt." [p. 11]

In hypnosis, an individual may become increasingly aware of his Umwelt (the environment around him), his Mitwelt (interpersonal relationships), and his Eigenwelt (the internal world of self). Cathexis refers to physical energy being lodged in or attaching itself to mental structures or processes. A deficiency of ego cathexis in the ego boundary results in feelings of estrangement and depersonalization characteristic of the schizoid personality and often of the pre-schizophrenic.

Because the concept of ego cathexis was developed by Paul Federn, the hypnotic manipulation of ego cathexis will be better understood after a brief discussion of Federn's Ego Psychology (1952).

Federn equated ego with ego feeling and distinguished a mental ego and a body ego. He contended that ego feeling is established by a psychic energy, which he called *ego cathexis.* If a part of my body is ego-cathected, or invested with this ego energy, it is a part of "I." My thoughts are also a part of me because they too are ego-cathected, or invested with this ego energy. If a thought broke through from unconsciousness without being invested with ego cathexis, I would sense it as object, therefore, a hallucination.

According to Federn, the ego is the only psychic institution which can be both subject and object, and the ego boundary is the peripheral sense organ of the ego. When internal stimuli include ego cathexis, they impinge on this ego boundary and are recognized as my thoughts. When external stimuli are devoid of ego cathexis, they strike the ego boundary and are sensed as perceptions of the external world.

Federn claimed that there are different ego states within the main boundaries of the ego, just as the United States is made up of many separate states, but all are part of one country. These ego states are all separated from each other, he theorized, but they can be activated by the transfer of ego cathexis from one to another.

As it is hypnotically suggested to the individual that ego cathexis flow in the direction of various ego boundaries, the boundaries that separate self from nonself, the individual's estrangement from his Umwelt and Mitwelt is reduced. Thus hypnotic techniques may be used to direct ego cathexis into the heart of self to counteract feelings of depersonalization and detachment which plague the schizoid personality and the preschizophrenic who find their Eigenwelts barren and suffer from what Kierkegaard has termed "the sickness unto death."

Several cases demonstrating the hypnotic manipulation of object and ego cathexes are presented here in order to illustrate the utilization of this technique. All of the cases were those of Watkins (1967).

The first case is an illustration of Umwelt alteration. The client, a middle-aged professional woman, complained of her difficulty in sensing a reality to the world. She found life unzestful and meaningless and did not receive sensations of tangible contact with objects. Her condition best fit the diagnostic category of schizoid personality.

During a session when she bitterly complained about her inability to sense any stimulating object, she was hypnotized and given the following suggestions: "All attention is being directed to your fingers. You do not need to experience sensations from any other part of your body. You will concentrate on your fingers, and they will tingle with aliveness. I am handing you now a pencil. You will feel this pencil, really feel it. It will be like an island of objective stimulation. It will seem so real, so vivid to your fingers." [p. 26]

The goal was to hypnotically direct all available ego cathexis into the finger part of the body ego and to energize that small part of the ego boundary. Its immediate success was apparent as the client burst into tears, exclaiming: "I really feel it. I really feel it. This is the first time in thirty years I have felt a pencil. I remember now how such things felt." [p. 26]

The next case is an example of Mitwelt alteration. The client was a young college professor referred for treatment of a reactive depression. There were multiple indications of his deep-seated resentment toward a dominating father, although he had so repressed the hostility that he was not conscious of its significance. In the words of Watkins, he had withdrawn object cathexis from his father's image and/or ego cathexis from that part of his ego boundary which was directed toward his father. Although interpretations were offered to him about his hostility both in hypnosis and in the conscious state, there was no change in his depressed condition. He heard the interpretations and had an intellectual acceptance of the hostility. One day he burst into the therapist's office and exclaimed, "My God, I do hate my father!" The cathectic illumination on the hated object had so increased that the hatred burst through repression with tremendous impact. With further elaboration and working through, the experimental insight would bring about a permanent change in his Mitwelt relationship toward a significant other.

The third case is an example of Eigenwelt alteration. A change in Eigenwelt, or self-concept, can alter body image, body, personality and the reactions of others, in that order. When asked in hypnosis to describe herself, the client, a heavy-set college student, burst into tears and stated that she was a fat, ugly, unlovable person. As her feelings of shame at her physical condition intensified, it was suggested to her that she obliterate any other experience except the present emotion and return to the time in her life when she first experienced it. She then relived an incident at the age of nine, when her mother told her that she was fat and ugly and would never be able to find a husband. She had internalized her mother's view and made it into a self-concept. She was given a combination of suggestions and interpretations which included the following:

> At the present time, you are overweight, but you are not an ugly and unlovable person . . . You accepted your mother's remark as

the absolute truth and believed that you were ugly and unlovable. Since you felt that people did not like you, it was so easy to take solace in eating. That's why you have gained so much weight. All of us here [this was part of a training session] think that you are a fine and attractive person. As you come to feel likewise, you will not have so much need to eat. In the meantime, whenever you eat your meals, you will tremendously enjoy the first bite of food. It will taste very good to you, and also the second. By the third bite you will begin to feel full, like one does after Thanksgiving dinner. You will enjoy the quality of the food and you will feel quite full and satisfied with very little quantity. As you lose weight, you will become increasingly encouraged and notice that people pay favorable attention to you and show that they like you. [p. 29]

The subject emerged from the hypnotic session all smiles and reported back later that day that she had eaten very little for lunch and that for the first time in many months she had lost her sense of anxiety and depression. Three weeks later, when reporting that she had lost eight pounds, she requested another hypnotic session to reemphasize the suggestions.

Repetition of such suggestions were continued until the loss of weight and the change to a happy disposition brought the more permanently reinforcing reactions from her friends and associates. As the derogatory self-image became decathected and the contradicting image of herself as an attractive and lovable person became invested with ego cathexis, her body adjusted to place it in harmony with this more constructive self-concept.

A number of hypnoanalytic techniques have been discussed here. These are by no means all of the techniques, but they are among the most frequently employed. There are indications with particular clients and at specific times within hypnoanalysis that each of these techniques would be appropriate. The decision as to when to employ a particular technique can only be made in the course of the analysis; the appropriateness of each technique with regard to the particular client and the phase of the analysis, as well as to the facility in utilizing the various techniques, can only be gained through extensive clinical experience. There are some cases in which the entire analysis would consist of the utilization of one technique, i.e., ideomotor questioning or age regression. On the other hand, cases are conceivable where it would be appropriate to employ a majority of hypnoanalytic techniques, even a number of them within one session. The proper use of these techniques will speed up an analysis, especially in those cases involving persons who find it difficult to verbalize while in hypnosis. Repressed material is often disclosed more readily, and there is a greater emotional participation on the part of the client. Since the employment of any of these uncovering techniques usually elicits a great deal of repressed material, which involves the expenditure of a large amount of psychic energy by the client, it is good to give the person twenty minutes to a half-hour of sleep after sessions in which these techniques have been used.

Part Five
Phases of
Hypnotherapy

Chapter 15.

The First Phase: History Taking

There is no way of arriving at the proper therapy for any emotionally disturbed person who comes for hypnotherapy except through diagnosis, and there is no proper way to diagnose except through a thorough history taking.

History taking is not merely the gathering of essential facts in order to support or disprove a hypothesis. It is an essential part of therapy. The dialogue during the history taking phase advances two essential factors inherent in the therapeutic process, namely, the growth of a strong trusting relationship between two persons and the gradual growth of insight, which arises from dialogue and encounter.

The matters about which a person elects to speak during the history taking phase are a selection from a much larger number of symptoms. The dominant mood of the person acts upon the association systems of the mind in such a way that memory becomes highly selective. Insofar as a person is caught up in an overpowering mood, it insists that he look at life in its own distorted way. Only those experiences which are in accordance with that mood are admitted to conscious recognition. The effect of this is to falsify the life history because of a memory bias.

The hypnotherapist must recognize that in listening to the un-structured history as related by an emotionally disturbed person, he is hearing a highly selective account of the past and most certainly a distorted one. When the client has had the opportunity to ventilate his feelings and rapport has been established, then a more structured history must be attempted. But initially it is important to let the client tell his story in his own way. A questionnaire for gathering historical data in a structured manner is included in Appendix A.

During the history taking phase, the client often has the tendency to hold back from disclosing the real nature of his worry. He feels the need to get to know the hypnotherapist better.

It is very important that the hypnotherapist be aware of the fact that the presenting symptom may be a screen symptom and may not at all coincide with the true problem. Screen symptoms may be factual (i.e., the person may be a compulsive hand washer but that isn't the real problem) and very convincing, and the hypnotherapist may believe that he has a full account of the person's difficulties. When hypnosis is going to be used in treatment, the danger lies in proceeding to hypnotic induction while the client is still consciously holding back. If a pattern of holding back is allowed to develop during the history taking, it is found to persist in induction. The client holds back, he doesn't let himself go, and hypnosis fails. The answer to the problem is the formation of rapport with plenty of time for adequate history taking.

The approach to history taking must always be leisurely. The client musn't be given any feeling of being rushed. History taking must always be thorough from the client's point of view. It should proceed easily and comfortably with a minimum of direct questions at the outset. The client should be casually brought to difficult areas and allowed to unburden himself in his own way. All the time, the therapist is developing the abandonment of the self, which is essential for hypnotic induction, hypnodiagnosis and analysis of the underlying disorder.

In the course of history taking, the hypnotherapist should ascertain the extent of every personal resource and strength. He should determine if there are any resources in the depths of the past on which to build in therapy.

In addition to evaluating the presented problem and ascertaining the extent of personal resources, history taking should include an evaluation of the client's psychological space and defense mechanisms.

Psychological space refers to a person's space for emotional movement. In determining the amount of psychological space available to a person, it is necessary to elicit the state of his defenses. The more he is using defense mechanisms, the more he is denying reality and the greater is the reduction in psychological space.

The most frequently encountered defense mechanisms will be presented at this time. *Repression* is purposeful but unconscious forgetting. This is probably the earliest defense available to the individual. *Suppression* is conscious, purposeful forgetting when the conflict can readily be recalled. *Regression* refers to a return to an earlier emotional level, which was more satisfying and at which the individual could adjust. *Rationalization* is the ascribing of acceptable motives to thoughts or behavior which really have other motives. *Projection* is attributing to another person or object thoughts or actions that are really one's own. *Introjection* refers to the turning of unacceptable tendencies against one's self. In *reaction formation,* the underlying impulse is so unacceptable or dangerous that overt behavior is directed in the opposite direction. *Denial* is conscious abregation. It is the simplest form of defense and is closely related to rationalization. In *isolation,* unacceptable impulses which appear in consciousness are separated from the remainder of the mental content. These are not all of the defenses against anxiety, but they do comprise the principal defense mechanisms seen in the major emotional disorders.

In addition to the foregoing, history taking restores continuity: it relates the present to the past and the past to the present.

Chapter 16.

The Second Phase: Training

During this phase of hypnotherapy, the client is trained in the development of visual imagery, in the achievement of his maximum depth of hypnosis, in the immediate reinduction of hypnosis by means of posthypnotic conditioning and in self-hypnosis. In addition, the client is given a number of ego strengthening suggestions and protective suggestions. The ego strengthening suggestions are repeated during each subsequent session after the induction of the hypnotic state.

The development of visual imagery may be accomplished by taking the client through each of the following steps:

1. In the waking state with his eyes closed, each client is asked to visualize, in his mind's eye, certain familiar objects, in this order: (a) a house, (b) a tree, (c) a person and (d) an animal. This step is continued until each stimulus has been achieved.

2. Following the attainment of image formation, the client is told: "Close your eyes and in your mind's eye visualize yourself as you are here, sitting in the chair *except the image of yourself has* his (her) eyes open.

3. At this point, the client is told to concentrate on the image and that all of the therapist's comments will be directed toward the client's *image* and *not* toward the client.

4. Then, a simple ocular-fixation technique is described and related to the eyelid closure of the image. Close clinical observation

of the client will reveal subtle response patterns, directly indicating the associative effect upon him. The client may be asked to confirm eyelid closure in the image, although often his own straining to open his eyelids will reveal the situation.

5. The next step involves moving directly into the induction relationship with the client. The initial induction technique and the accompanying suggestions should be determined by the nature of the client's defense. If the client appears to be relaxed, it is best to start with a progressive relaxation induction technique; if he is tense, then it is best to start with the tension-relaxation induction technique or arm levitation. If the client accepts the initial suggestions, then the hypnotic operator can proceed with the particular induction technique being used. However, if the client shows sustained defenses, then the hypnotic operator should proceed with the dynamic method of induction.

After the hypnotic state has been induced, the operator should proceed to train the subject to reach his maximum depth of hypnosis. It is a good practice to incorporate a deepening procedure into the induction technique. For example, if you are using an arm levitation technique, tell the subject that with each motion of the arm upward, he is going deeper and deeper into relaxation. Also, you may preface each step of the induction procedure with such phrases as, "If you really want to go deeper, you will take a deep breath." Such suggestions effectively motivate deepening of the hypnotic state.

Although a light or medium stage of hypnosis is suitable for purposes of physical relaxation and hypnotic suggestions for ego strengthening, desensitization and other methods of symptom removal, somnambulism is essential for most types of hypnoanalytic work, and therefore the hypnotic operator should know how to achieve this state. The most effective procedure for achieving somnambulism is by the induction of graded responses. This method involves deepening the hypnotic state by the application of a series of graduated steps, each being slightly more difficult than the last. A successful response to each of these in turn will progressively increase the subject's suggestibility and pave the way for the next step.

The following steps should be followed precisely; if they are, the majority of subjects will be capable of achieving somnambulism.

1. First, ask the subject to take three deep breaths, holding each breath for the count of four, opening the eyes wide when inhaling, closing them when exhaling.

2. Give the suggestion of eyelid heaviness each time the eyelids open.

3. Ask the subject to let his eyelids remain closed after exhaling for the third time.

4. Then ask the subject to relax the muscles around his eyes to the point where the eyelids just won't open.

5. Tell the subject that when he feels that his eyelids are completely relaxed, he is to try to open them, but that if they are completely relaxed they won't open (eyelid catalepsy).

6. When eyelid catalepsy has been achieved, ask the subject to send the complete relaxation he has in his eyelids throughout his entire body, from the top of his head down to the tips of his toes.

7. Then tell the subject that in a moment he is going to be asked to open his eyelids, and when he closes them again, he will be three times more relaxed than he is now.

8. Then ask the subject to open his eyelids and then to close them and to feel the increased relaxation throughout his entire body.

The following steps are for the induction of arm heaviness:

9. Place the subject's arm on the arm of the chair.

10. Stroke the subject's arm gently from the shoulder to the wrist.

11. Give the suggestion that as you stroke, the subject begins to feel a feeling of heaviness in his arm.

12. Give the suggestion that the feeling of heaviness is increasing with every stroke of your hand . . . just as heavy as if the arm were in a cast from the shoulder to the wrist.

13. Give the suggestion that as you continue to stroke the subject's arm, he can feel it pressing down more firmly on the arm of the chair.

14. As you say this, gradually increase the pressure of your own hand as you stroke the subject's arm.

15. Give the suggestion that in a few moments the subject's arm will feel so very heavy that when you pick it up by the wrist . . . and let go . . . it will drop limply into his lap.

16. Give the suggestion that as his hand drops limply into his lap, he will sink into a much deeper state of hypnosis.

17. Test the response by lifting the subject's arm by the wrist with the thumb and middle finger, raising the arm several feet in the air.

18. Let go of the arm by releasing your thumb and finger.

19. Restore the arm to normal by telling the subject that as you stroke his arm in the opposite direction . . . he will notice that all feelings of heaviness are leaving his arm.

20. Tell the subject that all feelings of heaviness have passed away completely and that his level of hypnosis has become even deeper.

The following steps are for the induction of automatic movements:

21. Instruct subject to place his elbow on the arm of the chair, with arm upwards and fingers pointing toward the ceiling.

22. Take the subject's arm by the wrist with the thumb and middle finger.

23. Move subject's arm slowly . . . backwards and forwards.

24. As you slowly move subject's arm backwards and forwards, ask him to imagine that a piece of cord is tied around his wrist . . . and that someone at each end of the cord is pulling his arm . . . first backwards . . . then forwards.

25. Ask subject to continue to picture that piece of cord tied around his wrist . . . pulling his arm slowly . . . backwards . . . and forwards; and that as he does so, he will find that when you release his wrist it will feel as if that piece of cord is still tied to it . . . still pulling his arm . . . backwards . . . and forwards.

26. Tell subject that his arm will go on moving . . . entirely on its own . . . backwards and forwards . . . until you tell it to stop.

27. Tell subject that he won't try to make it move and he won't try to stop it from moving, but will just let it go on moving on its own . . . quite automatically . . . backwards and forwards . . . until you tell it to stop.

28. When the arm is moving freely, tell subject that his level of hypnosis is becoming deeper, timing this so that you repeat the word 'deeper' on each alternate forward movement of his arm.

29. After six automatic movements forwards and backwards, tell the subject to stop and put his arm back on the arm of the chair.

30. Tell subject that as his arm touches the arm of the chair, he is falling into an even deeper state of hypnosis.

The following steps are for the induction of amnesia for numbers:

31. Ask the subject to visualize himself in front of a blackboard and to visualize the blackboard tray with chalk and erasers.

32. Then ask him to pick up a piece of chalk and to write the numbers one to ten on the blackboard.

33. Then ask him to erase all of the even numbers and that as he does that, the even numbers are being erased from his mind.

34. Then ask him to count from one to ten.

35. Then ask the subject to pick up the piece of chalk again and to write in all of the even numbers again.

36. Then ask him to count from one to ten.

Then, achieve somnambulism with the eyes open by the following steps for the induction of glove anesthesia with the eyes open:

37. Stroke the subject's right hand and tell him that as you stroke his hand, it is going to become more and more numb.

38. Ask the subject to imagine that his hand is submerged in a bucket of ice water, and that it is surrounded by ice.

39. Then tell the subject that you are going to pinch his left hand.

40. Pinch his left hand and ask if he feels any pain.

41. Then tell the subject that you are going to pinch his right hand.

42. Pinch his right hand and ask if he feels anything.

43. Tell the subject that in a moment you are going to ask him to open his eyes and that as he does the numbness in his right hand will be three times greater than it is now.

44. Ask the subject to open his eyes and look down at his right hand.

45. Ask the subject to take his left hand and give his right hand a good pinch.

46. Ask the subject if he feels anything.

47. Tell the subject to let his eyes close again and as he does, suggest that he will go into a much deeper state of hypnosis.

48. Then stroke the subject's right hand and tell him that as you stroke his right hand, all of the feeling and warmth is returning to it and that now it feels the same as his left hand.

Somnambulism with the eyes open is necessary for the utilization of a number of hypnoanalytic techniques, such as hypnoplasty and hypnography.

The therapist now proceeds with the induction of posthypnotic conditioning. This enables him to immediately induce a deep state of hypnosis upon signal in future sessions, without the time-consuming need of repeating a lengthy induction and deepening procedure.

With the subject still in hypnosis, proceed with the following steps:

1. Tell the subject that in a moment, you will wake him up by counting from five to one.

2. Tell the subject that at the count of one, he will open his eyes . . . feeling wonderfully refreshed as a result of this deep state of relaxation.

3. Tell the subject that after he has opened his eyes and returned to the normal waking state, you will talk to him for a minute or two.

4. Then ask the subject to sit back comfortably in his chair and look straight into your eyes.

5. Tell the subject that the moment he hears you say *relax,* his eyes will close immediately and he will drift immediately into a state of hypnosis at least as deep as the one he is in now.

6. While he is looking into your eyes, say "RELAX!"

7. Bring the subject out of hypnosis in the following manner: "In a moment when I count from five to one . . . with every number I count . . . you will feel your whole body becoming lighter . . . and feel yourself becoming more alert. At the count of one . . . your eyes will open . . . and you will be wide awake and alert. You will feel completely refreshed as a result of this complete physical and mental relaxation. Five . . . four . . . three . . . two . . . one!"

8. As soon as the subject opens his eyes, ask him about his feelings during hypnosis and discuss his reactions.

9. Then ask him to sit back in his chair and look straight into your eyes.

10. While the subject is looking into your eyes, say to him firmly, "RELAX!"

11. If the eyelids do not close immediately, repeat the suggestion much more firmly, once or twice if necessary.

12. Then proceed to consolidate this conditioning for all future occasions in the following manner: "From now on . . . whenever you are sitting in that chair . . . all that I will have to do is to ask you to sit back comfortably in the chair and look straight at me. While you are looking at me . . . I will say, 'RELAX!' And from now on . . . whenever you hear me say . . . 'RELAX' . . . your eyelids will always close immediately . . . and you will always go immediately . . . into a deep state of hypnosis . . . at least as deep as the one you are in now. And that is exactly what is going to happen when you come to see me the next time. After our preliminary talk . . . I will ask you to sit back comfortably in your chair . . . and look straight at me. While you are looking at me . . . I will say . . . 'RELAX!' Your eyelids will close immediately . . . and you will go immediately into a deep state of hypnosis . . . at least as deep as the one you are in now."

The therapist should then proceed to train the client in self-hypnosis, using the technique developed by Dr. Peter Lindner (1965). The following steps should be followed precisely.

1. The subject is told to choose one finger from both hands and to stiffen that finger.

2. Then he is told to count to three, and to make the finger more and more stiff with the idea in mind that when he gets to THREE, he will not be able to bend it.

3. Then say the following to the subject: "Now, lets start counting. ONE . . . make the fingers more rigid . . . TWO . . . more rigid yet . . . make them as rigid as a piece of steel . . . all right, now you are ready for the last number . . . THREE . . . make them even stiffer . . . so stiff and rigid that you just cannot bend them . . . you can try to bend them, but they won't bend at all . . . that's right, you have made them so completely rigid that they just won't bend. . . ."

4. Then say: "Now, as I count to three once more, they will slowly bend again and feel perfectly normal. ONE . . . bending a little . . . TWO . . . let them bend some more . . . and . . . THREE . . . and now the fingers are completely flexible and normal—just as they were before you started."

5. Then ask the subject to repeat the rigid finger maneuver once more with one slight change in the procedure. After the fingers are stiff, tell him to suggest to himself: "As my fingers bend, my eyes will close, so that by the end of my third count, my eyes will be shut and my eyelids will be so relaxed and limp that they will not work or open *unless I let the tension come back into them by blinking.* I want this to happen, I expect it to happen, and I will watch it happen."

6. Tell the subject that as soon as the fingers are rigid, he is to open his eyes wide and not blink them from then on, because he is going to condition himself to rouse from the hypnotic state by blinking his eyelids.

7. Tell the subject to let his eyelids close slowly without blinking.

8. After the eyelids have closed, tell the subject to let his eyelids develop a progressive feeling of relaxation, until they seem so relaxed that it is just too much effort to make them work or open.

9. Then tell him to lock his mind around the idea that his eyelids are so relaxed that they will not work or open. Then tell him to test them to make sure that they won't work.

10. Then tell the subject to blink his eyelids and feel them pop open.

11. Tell the subject to send that complete relaxation in the eyelid muscles all the way throughout his body to his feet.

12. Tell the subject to imagine himself like a rag doll, with arms and legs limp and dangling down, as he sends the relaxation through his body.

13. Then tell the subject to imagine that if someone were to pick up his arm and drop it, it would just flop down like a wet dishcloth.

14. Tell the subject then that he has entered into a state of hypnosis, but that when he is first learning to enter this state, he should also employ a simple deepening technique, such as repeating to himself the following: "In a moment, I am going to blink my eyes and they will open. I will then close them again, and as I close them the next time, I will find myself three times more deeply relaxed than I am right now."

15. Then tell the subject to proceed as planned, and that as he closes his eyelids, he is to let himself feel a very pleasant surge of relaxation, which he is to allow to travel down to his toes.

16. Then tell the subject to compound the suggestion once more, while thinking the following thoughts: "I will open my eyelids once more by blinking them. But when I close them the next time, I will be twice as relaxed as I am now. I will feel so completely relaxed that every last bit of tension in my body will have disappeared. I will just let myself be covered by a blanket of relaxation from head to toe."

17. In conclusion, tell the subject that as he repeats this procedure daily, he will be able to achieve greater depths of hypnosis each time.

The therapist should then give ego-strengthening suggestions. The ego-strengthening technique presented here was developed by Dr. John Hartland (1965, 1971). Hartland postulated the following principle, upon which the subsequent development of the ego-strengthening technique was based:

> In all cases, direct symptom removal will be most successful . . .
> if, at each and every session, it is preceded by a sequence of simple psychotherapeutic suggestions designed to remove tension, anxiety and apprehension, and to restore the patient's confidence in himself and his ability to cope with his problems.

The ego-strengthening technique has been carefully constructed in accordance with the following principles: (1) Repetition is often achieved by expressing the same fundamental idea in several different ways, thereby avoiding excessive monotony. (2) Some words and phrases are stressed because of their importance and significance to the patient himself. (3) Other words are stressed with the sole purpose of emphasizing the rhythm of the whole delivery. (4) The interpolation of appropriate pauses in conjunction with the stressing of key words establishes a rhythmical quality to the delivery, similar to the beat of a metronome.

Hartland has found the ego-strengthening technique to be equally valuable either as a prelude to direct symptom removal or hypnoanalysis. Constant repetition at the beginning of every therapeutic session strengthens the ego to such an extent that it not only renders the symptoms more vulnerable to direct suggestion, but will often enable a client to cooperate subsequently in a hypnoanalytical situation that he was formerly unable to face.

Begin the ego-strengthening with the following approach:

"Every day . . . you will become physically *stronger* and *fitter:* You will become *more alert . . . more wide awake . . . more energetic.* You will become *much less easily tired . . . much less easily fatigued . . . much less easily depressed . . . much less easily discouraged.*

"Every day . . . you will become *so deeply interested in whatever you are doing . . . so deeply interested in whatever is going on . . . that your mind will become much less preoccupied with yourself . . . and you will become much less conscious of yourself . . . and your own feelings.*

"Every day . . . *your nerves will become stronger and steadier . . . your mind will become calmer and clearer . . . more composed . . . more placid . . . more tranquil.* You will become *much less easily worried . . . much less easily agitated . . . much less fearful and apprehensive . . . much less easily upset.*

"You will be able to *think more clearly . . .* you will be able to *concentrate more easily . . . your memory will improve . . .* and you will be able to *see things in their true perspective . . . without magnifying them . . . without allowing them to get out of proportion.*

"Every day . . . you will feel *a greater feeling of personal well-being . . . a greater feeling of personal safety and security . . .* than you have felt for a long, long time.

"Every day . . . *you* will become . . . and *you* will remain . . . *more and more completely relaxed . . . and less tense each day . . . both mentally and physically . . .* even when you are no longer with me.

"And, *as* you become . . . and, *as* you remain . . . *more relaxed . . . and less tense each day . . . so* you will develop *much more confidence in yourself, much* more confidence in your ability to *do*

... *not* only what you *have* to do each day ... but, *much* more confidence in your ability to do whatever you *ought* to be able to do ... *without fear of consequences* ... *without fear of failure* ... *without unnecessary anxiety* ... *without uneasiness.*

"Because of this ... every day ... you will feel *more and more independent* ... *more able to stick up for yourself* ... *to stand upon your own feet* ... *to hold your own* ... *no matter how difficult or trying things may be.*

"And, because all these things will begin to happen ... *exactly* as I tell you they will happen, you will begin to feel *much happier* ... *much more contented* ... *much more cheerful* ... *much more optimistic* ... *much less discouraged* ... *much less easily depressed.*"

Conclude the session by reassuring the client with the following protective suggestions:

1. You will never be able to be hypnotized by anyone but a qualified practitioner.

2. You will never be able to be taken advantage of in any way while in hypnosis.

3. You will never be able to be hypnotized unless you want to be hypnotized; you cannot be hypnotized against your will.

4. You will never be able to be hypnotized while at the wheel of an automobile, while operating any moving machinery, or in any situation in which it may be dangerous to you.

5. Should you be hypnotized and should an emergency situation arise which requires your immediate attention, such as a fire in the building, you would immediately become alert and clear-headed and be able to handle the situation capably and efficiently.

6. Should you feel that you need any other suggestion to protect you while in hypnosis, that suggestion is given to you and takes full and complete effect upon you just the same as if I had said it.

7. In addition to the six protective suggestions I have given you, from this moment on whenever I say the word *relax* to you when you are in this office and sitting in that chair for the purpose of hypnotic treatment, you will immediately drop into a deep hypnotic state, even deeper than the one you are in now. Your eyes will close, all of your muscles will relax completely, your mind will relax completely, and you will continue to go deeper with every breath you

take until I bring you out of hypnosis. The word *relax* in ordinary conversation will neither disturb you nor produce a hypnotic state.

The client is brought out of the hypnotic state by repeating the following:

"In a moment I am going to count backwards from five to one. With each number that I count, your whole body will feel lighter and lighter and you will become more and more alert. At the count of one, your eyes will open and you will be wide awake and alert, feeling very relaxed . . . five . . . feeling lighter and lighter throughout your entire body . . . four . . . becoming more and more alert . . . three . . . lighter throughout your whole body and much more alert . . . two . . . and . . . one . . . eyes open . . . wide awake . . .very alert . . . and completely relaxed and refreshed . . . both physically and mentally."

Chapter 17.

The Third Phase: Hypnodiagnosis

The hypnotherapist who has taken a thorough history and been an attentive listener during the first phase of therapy will be able to hazard a diagnosis of the nature of the problem. However, this is only part of the diagnosis, the part based upon the presenting symptoms. During the hypnodiagnostic phase, we are concerned with arriving at the underlying diagnosis.

In the hypnodiagnostic phase, the disorder should always be assessed against the psychological background of the individual. To do this, it is necessary to seek the answers to the following questions: (1) Why did this person become emotionally ill in the first place? (2) What kind of a person is he? and (3) Why did he develop this particular disorder?

During the hypnodiagnostic phase, there are a number of specific techniques that can be utilized to help the hypnotherapist arrive at an accurate assessment of the client's internal conflicts. The following hypnodiagnostic techniques will be discussed: scene visualization, the association technique, and ideomotor questioning.

The neurotic conscience of the emotionally disturbed person, on the one hand, keeps a constant eye on the repressed destructive emotions, keeping them firmly under cover; on the other hand, to complete the deception and cover up all traces of the destructive impulses which have been buried alive, leans over backwards to develop a character-type (i.e., neurotic ego ideal) which is precisely

147

the opposite of the repressed emotions. This is what is meant by the bipolar nature of neurotic conflict.

Scene Visualization

The bipolar nature of neurotic conflict can be utilized in hypnodiagnosis by means of bipolarization questions, which are a form of the scene visualization technique. The bipolarization questions to be presented were developed by Dr. Joseph Shorr (1972). The questions should be asked while the client is in hypnosis. One bipolarization question is to ask the client to imagine himself turning around 180 degrees and then imagine opening his eyes and seeing anything at all. Then he is asked what he sees. The methods to uncover the 180 degree variations are infinite. The client may be asked to imagine two large boxes and then asked what person he imagines in each box. A good way to help the client arrive at his own awareness of his conflicts is to ask him to imagine two different animals, give an adjective to each, assign a verb to each, have each animal say something to each other; then he is asked what would happen if these two animals were in conflict with each other and whether the conflict between the two animals has anything to do with his own conflict.

Another use of scene visualization for assessing how the client feels about himself, his conflicts and what he will do about it is to ask him to imagine that he is on top of a mountain and also on a ledge below. Then he is told that the top self lowers a rope to the bottom self; he is then asked what will happen. This method, also developed by Shorr (1972), provides the hypnotherapist and the client with the client's attitude towards allowing help. The client's stake in maintaining his neurotic solution can be examined by means of such an imaginary situation.

Another very effective use of scene visualization is the five-minute life history developed by Shorr (1972). The client is asked in a time limit of five minutes to grow up from a baby, in a baby's room. He will invariably recall the significant life events that are emotionally charged for him and he will indicate how he has been defined by others.

There are a number of additional variations on scene visualization. The client might be asked to observe a stage in a theater and report the scene that appears when the curtains are drawn, or to turn on an imaginary TV set to a program that will reveal an important aspect of his problem, or to open a door upon a secret room that contains forgotten images of the past. Scene visualization can also be used in conjunction with the idea association technique by asking the client to visualize the word-stimuli or sentence stem given and to give his thoughts to the visualization.

IDEA ASSOCIATION

The idea association technique is an effective method for uncovering the more complex emotional blockages. The client is either given a word and asked to respond by saying the first thing that enters his mind, or a sentence stem and asked to complete the sentence with the first thing that comes to mind. Through these probes with word stimuli and sentence stems, the chief complexes often emerge clearly.

Obviously, the number of word stimuli and sentence stems that can allow a person to become aware of his internal conflicts is infinite. The idea association technique puts the hypnotherapist in touch with the inner conflicts, needs, fantasies, aspirations, attitudes and adjustment difficulties of the client.

A diagnostic instrument that makes use of the idea association technique is included in Appendix B. *The Hypnodiagnostic Association Test* is administered to the client while he is in hypnosis.

The hypnodiagnostic techniques presented thus far are techniques for uncovering attitudes that may be either conscious, subconscious, or a mixture of both. The next hypnodiagnostic technique to be discussed, ideomotor questioning, elicits information directly from the subconscious mind.

IDEOMOTOR QUESTIONING

Ideomotor questioning may be used to gain significant information that is either not as easily available or not available at all by other more conventional means. In discussing this technique, Cheek and LeCron (1968), a physician and clinical psychologist, stated: "We regard this as the most valuable of all uncovering methods. In one session, more information can be learned than in many hours of free association, unless there is strong resistance." [p. 85]

The ideomotor questioning technique has been described by LeCron (1954), Cheek (1960), LeBaron (1964) and Denniston (1968). Ideomotor activity refers to the involuntary capacity of muscles to respond instantaneously to thoughts, feelings and ideas.

This technique consists of wording questions so that they can be answered either affirmatively or negatively. This sets up a code of signals, which the subconscious mind utilizes in replying. These signals are subconsciously controlled movements of the client's fingers.

Before beginning the ideomotor questioning, the hypnotherapist should explain to the client that the inner part of the mind controls all of the involuntary functions of the body, such as breathing, heart beat and regulation of body temperature. It is much easier for the inner mind to control movements of the fingers than to control and regulate the muscles involved in breathing. Then the client should be told that his inner mind is going to be asked some questions and that the answers will help to get to the heart of the problem. He may also be told that the inner or subconscious mind is like a tape recorder: it is a storehouse of every experience, memory or thought that a person has had since birth.

When employing ideomotor questioning, the client is told, while in hypnosis, that the forefingers and thumbs are under the control of his subconscious mind. The subconscious mind is directed to reply to questions by lifting the right forefinger to indicate *yes,* the left forefinger to indicate *no,* the right thumb to signal *don't know,* and the left thumb for *refusal to answer.* Leading questions such as "Don't you think?" should be avoided. When wording questions, it is essential to make the meaning clear and unambiguous: the subconscious takes everything literally. In ideomotor questioning, always consider carefully whether or not it is safe to bring repressed conflicts into consciousness, for some might be intolerable and overwhelming. "Is it all right for you to know the reason for this?" and "Is it all right for you to remember?" are questions that should be asked. If the reply is negative, no attempt should be made to delve further at the time.

A copy of the *Ideomotor Response Questionnaire,* with instructions to the client, is included in Appendix C.

These hypnodiagnostic techniques enhance each other as they are combined and interwoven. Even singly, they are valuable, but in combination, the whole is much greater than each of its parts. It has already been shown how scene visualization may be used in conjunction with the idea association technique. Another example of combining techniques would be a case where, if the client is not responding to ideomotor questioning, the hypnotherapist shifts to scene visualization and asks the client to imagine a blackboard in front of him. Then he is asked to visualize an imaginary hand writing words or a sentence on the blackboard in white chalk. Often this will produce an important clue.

Age regression can be an invaluable aid in hypnodiagnosis as well as in history taking. By age regressing the hypnotized person back to the time of onset of the disorder, a more accurate and complete history and diagnosis of the disorder can be obtained than by merely asking the client to recall the onset and progression of the disorder from memory alone.

Other hypnodiagnostic techniques include figure drawing, automatic writing, and the use of projective tests in conjunction with hypnosis.

The use of any hypnodiagnostic technique requires a great deal of flexibility and imagination on the part of the hypnotherapist. It cannot be emphasized too strongly that these techniques should not be used in a cookbook fashion.

Although we designate this as the hypnodiagnostic phase, diagnosis should be an ongoing aspect of hypnotherapy. To some extent the individual is always rewriting his history to serve the adjustment needs of the present and the future. Whether the data derived during the hypnodiagnostic phase are unique, or whether they confirm, contradict or confuse, it is the task of the hypnotherapist to create a new synthesis of meaning that will take them into account at least as current operative fantasies, along with all the other information derived from clinical interaction.

Chapter 18.

The Fourth Phase: Teaching

When reconstructive hypnoanalysis is the treatment choice, several sessions should be spent in teaching the client various hypnoanalytic processes that will be utilized during the analytic phase. The client must be impressed with the fact that this phase of therapy is devoted exclusively to teaching hypnoanalytic procedures and that discussion of symptoms and conflicts must be avoided.

At the end of the teaching phase, the client should possess the following capabilities necessary for the progress of the analysis:

(1) He should be able to carry out posthypnotic suggestions with ease and rapidity, including posthypnotic amnesia.

(2) He should be able to revert memorially to former scenes and places.

(3) He should be able to dream upon suggestion.

(4) He should be able to either expand or condense time upon suggestion.

(5) He should be able to experience positive hallucinations with the eyes open while remaining in a deep state of hypnosis; and

(6) He should be able to write or draw automatically upon suggestion with the eyes open while remaining deeply hypnotized.

Methods of producing each of these hypnoanalytic procedures will now be presented.

Posthypnotic Amnesia

I use the chalkboard technique to teach posthypnotic amnesia. With the client in the somnambulistic state, proceed with the following steps:

1. Ask the subject to imagine that he can see a chalkboard . . . and that you are standing in front of it with a piece of chalk in your hand.

2. Tell the subject that as soon as he can see it quite clearly, to let you know by lifting his right index finger.

3. As soon as the subject's finger rises, tell him that as he watches the chalkboard, he will see you writing his home address with the chalk.

4. Tell him that as soon as he can see his home address on the chalkboard, to lift his right index finger.

5. After the subject's finger rises, tell him that as he continues to look at the chalkboard, he can see that you have taken an eraser and are erasing the address from the chalkboard.

6. Give the suggestion that as his home address is being erased from the chalkboard, it is also being erased from his mind.

7. Tell the subject that as soon as he can see that his home address has disappeared and that the chalkboard is clear and blank, to lift his right index finger.

8. Then tell the subject that in a few moments, when you bring him out of hypnosis, he will not be able to remember his home address . . . until you touch him on the right shoulder. Then he will remember.

9. Then bring the subject out of hypnosis by counting backwards from five to one, giving the suggestion that with every number you count, he will feel lighter and lighter and more and more wide awake and alert.

10. Tell the subject that when you reach the count of one, his eyelids will open, and he will be wide awake, alert and refreshed.

11. Tell the subject that when you ask him for his home address, he will not remember it . . . until you touch him on the right shoulder. Then he will remember his home address.

12. Then count from five to one.

13. After the subject opens his eyes, ask him what his home address is.

14. After the subject tries for approximately 30 seconds to recall his home address, touch him on the right shoulder, whereupon he will remember his address.

REVIVIFICATION

Revivification involves an actual return to an earlier age, with a true reliving of the events at that particular time. This is true age regression: in this altered state of consciousness, the client is able to recapture memories and relive events that have long been forgotten.

In teaching revivification, proceed with the following steps:

1. Tell the subject that while he is in this deep state of hypnosis, time no longer matters.
2. Then tell him that he will be able to go back quite easily to an earlier period of life.
3. Give the suggestion that he feels that he is gradually getting smaller . . . that his arms and legs are getting smaller . . . that his whole body is getting smaller.
4. Give the suggestion that when he goes back to an earlier period of his life, you will be someone he knows and likes.
5. Give the suggestion to the subject that he is gradually going back to the time of his fifth birthday.
6. Tell the subject that in a few moments he will feel that he is five years old again, and that it is his birthday.
7. Ask the subject to let you know as soon as he feels that he is exactly five years old by lifting his right index finger.
8. As soon as the subject lifts his right index finger, he can be questioned as to who he is, where he is, how old he is, what he is doing and what presents he has received.

DREAMING UPON SUGGESTION

The client can be taught to develop the ability to dream in response to hypnotic suggestion. I have found the approach of Hartland (1966) to be very effective in this regard.

In teaching the client to dream upon suggestion, proceed with the following steps:

1. Tell the subject that he is now so deep in hypnosis, that in a few moments, when you tell him to dream . . . he will dream.
2. Then tell the subject that he will dream that he is performing whatever action you tell him to dream about.
3. Tell him that he will be able to picture himself quite clearly and see himself quite vividly . . . in his own mind . . . carrying out whatever action you have told him to dream about.

4. Then tell the subject that he is going to dream that he is drinking a glass of water.

5. Repeat the suggestion that he is going to dream that he is drinking a glass of water.

6. Ask the subject to show you what he is dreaming.

In a positive response, the subject's hand will move slowly upwards and perform the action that has been suggested.

POSITIVE HALLUCINATIONS

Positive hallucinations involving any of the senses can be produced in a somnambulistic subject by appropriate suggestions. In somnambulism, the eyes may be opened without affecting the depth of hypnosis.

Positive hallucinations have therapeutic applications in hypnoanalysis. Crystal gazing in hypnosis is a form of visual hallucination. When instructed to gaze into the crystal, the subject will see and describe scenes that arise from his own internal conflicts. This technique is frequently used in hypnoanalysis.

With the subject in the somnambulistic state, positive hallucinations with the eyes open may be produced by following the method developed by Hartland (1966). Proceed with the following steps:

1. With his eyes still closed, tell the subject that you want him to visualize in his mind's eye that you are holding a glass of water in front of his eyes.

2. Tell him to notice that it is colorless, but that as he continues to watch it . . . it gradually becomes pinker and pinker . . . and then changes to a reddish color.

3. Ask the subject to let you know as soon as he can see the color changing by lifting his right index finger.

4. As soon as the right index finger rises, tell the subject that in a moment he will open his eyes but that he will not wake from this deep state of hypnosis.

5. Then tell the subject that his eyes will open slowly but that he will remain in a deep state of hypnosis . . . even though his eyes are wide open.

6. Then tell the subject that he will see everything that you point out to him.

7. Give the suggestion that when he opens his eyes, he will notice that you are holding a glass of clear water in front of his eyes.

8. Tell the subject that as he watches it, he will see the color of the water slowly becoming pinker and pinker . . . until it becomes quite red . . . just as it did when his eyes were closed.

9. Ask the subject to open his eyelids slowly . . . wider and wider.

10. Give the suggestion that as he looks at the glass of water in your hand, he will see the color changing . . . first to pink . . . then to red.

11. Ask the subject to let you know as soon as he sees the color changing by lifting his right index finger.

12. As soon as the subject's finger rises, tell him to continue to look at the glass of water, and that when the color has changed to red, to let you know by lifting his right index finger.

13. Once this has occurred, the subject can be told that as he looks at your desk, he will see a burning candle in a candlestick.

14. Then he is told to go over to the desk and blow out the candle.

AUTOMATIC WRITING

This technique is of value when a situation in hypnoanalysis arises that can be solved by the expression of a single word or phrase. The hypnotized client will often write down ideas which he will not or cannot express verbally.

In teaching automatic writing, proceed with the following steps:

1. Have the hypnotized subject seated at a table.

2. Then induce automatic movement of the hand and arm used for writing.

3. Then place a pencil in the subject's hand and a blank piece of paper before him on the table.

4. Give the suggestion that his hand and arm feel as if they are completely detached from the rest of his body.

5. It is then suggested that his hand will begin to write quite automatically so that he will not be aware of what he is writing.

6. The idea of automatic activity should be stressed in the following manner: "Your hand works automatically. It writes it down. It writes it down automatically."

Chapter 19.

The Fifth Phase:
Treatment or Analysis

By the conclusion of the diagnostic phase, a treatment plan has been formulated. The type of hypnotherapy to be utilized is determined by the nature of the problem, the personality structure of the client, the client's level of motivation and his ability as a hypnotic subject. If one of the hypnotherapeutic types of hypnotic treatment is indicated, then this phase is referred to as the treatment phase; if one of the hypnoanalytic types is called for, then it is called the analytic phase.

The chapters on hypnoidal therapy and direct hypnotherapy describe what takes place during the treatment phase. The following is a description of the analytic phase during reconstructive hypnoanalysis.

During the analytic phase, the therapist is concerned with uncovering events that produced a sufficient threat to the client's survival (being) or self-worth (well-being) that an area of ontological anxiety was established in the client's mind; his aim is to enable the client to focus on the events in order to release the negative emotion connected with each, to replace the negative emotional content with positive emotional content and to help the client to discard conflicting and unrealistic self-models.

The emotionally powerful incident by which the individual is first sensitized is referred to as the Initial Sensitizing Event (Boswell, 1961). This event has usually been repressed from consciousness.

159

"Psychological antibodies" build up against the Initial Sensitizing Event but no symptoms appear. A second emotionally powerful event triggers the symptom into production as the "psychological antigen" meets the "psychological antibodies" of the sensitized organism. This event is referred to as the Symptom Producing Event. The Symptom Intensifying Event produces still further difficulties. There may be more than one Symptom Intensifying Event.

As was mentioned earlier, one of the primary objectives in the analytic phase is to uncover the events and to remove the negative emotions connected with each. There are a number of techniques which may be used for this purpose. The uncovering techniques utilized depend to a large extent on the client's development as a hypnotic subject and on the type of disorder and its severity. These techniques stimulate unconscious mental activity of a constructive nature.

In the analytic phase, we are first of all concerned with a catharsis (i.e., a release into conscious awareness of repressed experiences from the subconscious mind) of traumatic events which gave rise to the disorder. This is accomplished by the utilization of uncovering or reentry methods. The uncovering hypnoanalytic techniques that I have found to be most revealing of unconscious material and most helpful in overcoming resistance to the recall of unconscious traumatic material are described in detail in the chapter on reconstructive hypnoanalysis.

After the client has recalled, by means of the uncovering techniques, the traumatic incidents (Initial Sensitizing Event, Symptom Producing Event, and Symptom Intensifying Events) that led to the formation of his disorder, he is helped to focus his feelings and to confront the perpetrators of his conflict. The focusing techniques leading to abreaction are many. The following are those that I have found to be most useful: The Impossible Scream; I Am Not—I Am; Your Face in My Hands—My Face in Your Hands; Eyeball-to-Eyeball; and Transforming the Eyes of the Other. These techniques were developed by Shorr (1972) and are described in detail in his excellent book.

THE IMPOSSIBLE SCREAM

After the client has recalled the traumatic event, he may be asked to imagine the significant person (i.e., father or mother) in front of him and to tell the therapist what would be the most impossible thing to scream at that person. It is important to be as specific as possible in the impossible scream confrontation. It is necessary for the client to scream what will liberate, not just to scream anything. When the screaming is over, most persons report feeling free. The scream may have been literally waiting a lifetime for release.

I AM NOT—I AM

In this technique, the client is asked to imagine the person who is being confronted before him and to scream at the person, "I am not—; I am—!" The therapist should ask for as many pairs of nouns or adjectives as the client will offer. One client's responses were: "I am not a thing; I am a human being! I am not to be ignored; I am a person!"

YOUR FACE IN MY HANDS—MY FACE IN YOUR HANDS

A very effective technique for abreaction and liberation is to have the client imagine that he is holding his mother's face in his hands. The therapist may then ask: "What do you feel?" "What do you see?" "Now, say something to your mother." "What does she say to you?" Variations of holding the face can be made by reversing the self and other by having the parent hold the client's face or having the therapist hold the client's face. Any variation of this technique has as its purpose the focusing of the client's feelings and awareness toward conflict resolution.

EYEBALL-TO-EYEBALL

In this technique, there is a confrontation with the client standing as if he is standing eyeball-to-eyeball with the person who is the source of his problem. The Impossible Scream can be used in conjunction with this technique. The client is urged to acknowledge the anxiety he feels in relation to each of the traumatic events which have been uncovered, but accompanying the acknowledgment must be genuine feelings of relinquishment of the responsibility for the anxiety. Some liberating statements to the significant person may be: "I won't feel anxious anymore because you didn't come when I needed you." "I no longer feel that I am unworthy."

TRANSFORMING THE EYES OF THE OTHER

In applying this technique, the client is encouraged in his imagination to stare into the eyes of the person who he greatly fears and stare until he can feel that he is transforming the eyes of the other from negative to more positive feelings. If the client expresses anxiety over the condemning look of the other person, he should be urged to keep staring until he can transform the eyes so that they are not condemning him.

After all of the significant events of the past have been uncovered, and after the negative emotions connected with each event have been removed and replaced with positive ones, the therapist proceeds to the deeper aspects of analysis, that is, the dramatic analytic situation of the present. The first part of the analysis dealt with the uncovering of traumas or incidents of the past. It is the present, existential situation of the client, who is at a loss as to how to deal with conflicting and unworthy self-models, that concerns the therapist at this deeper level of analysis. A consideration of the various existing and conflicting models can be a rich and extremely valuable part of the analytic phase of treatment.

The multiplicity of models that prevent or obscure present self-recognition may be classified as follows: (1) what he believes he is (in which he overevaluates himself); (2) what he would like to be (idealized, unattainable models); (3) what he would like to appear to be to others; (4) the models of what others believe him to be; (5) models that others make of what they would like him to be, and (6) models that others evoke and produce in him.

Before working with the client on the specific ideal model in the hypnosynthesis phase, we need to make him aware of all these models, which may be conflicting and some of which are largely unconscious. This may be accomplished by means of the hypnoanalytic technique of hallucinated images of multiple crystal balls, developed by Milton Erickson (1958). The client is asked to visualize a series of crystal balls. Then he is told that he will see himself in each crystal ball as one of the images or models which prevent or obscure present self-recognition (i.e., "in the first crystal ball you will see an image of yourself as you believe you are; in the second crystal ball you will see an image of yourself as you would like to be, etc.").

Chapter 20.

The Sixth Phase:
Reeducation Synthesis

During this phase, the client is helped to realize that the symptom is unnecessary and an ineffectual method of satisfying his needs; he is helped to find adequate substitutes.

Reeducation involves integration of new life decisions and acquisition of skill in their practice, as well as a clarification of basic values, an inventory of life goals, and the achievement of imagery experience.

The client's symptom has served a number of purposes. It has defended him against anxiety; it has helped to structure his time; it has provided him with certain secondary gains; it has prevented him from doing certain things; and it has influenced the nature of his interpersonal relationships.

For example, if the client has had a drinking problem, the fact that he no longer drinks cannot be viewed as a cure and the end of therapy. A number of other questions must be asked and satisfactory answers found for those questions before therapy is complete. In what ways can he handle anxiety other than with alcohol? In what positive ways can he structure his time now that he is no longer drinking, fighting with his wife, etc.? Since most of his social interactions were while under the influence of alcohol, what skills does he need to learn in order to relate to people in positive ways? Since he was getting a great deal of attention, secondary gain and positive as well as negative reinforcement for his drinking, in what ways can he get positive reinforcement and recognition now that he is no longer drinking?

CLARIFICATION OF BASIC VALUES

The client is given a blank sheet of paper and is asked to answer the following questions (from James and Jongeward, 1971):

Who and what do I value?
Who and what do I live for?
Who and what would I die for?
What does my life mean to me now?
What could it mean?
What does my life mean to others now?
What is really important? [p. 276]

The client is then given another blank sheet of paper and asked to write the following at the top of the sheet: "These Are My Basic Values." Then the client is asked to list the five things he values most in his life. He should then rate the values in order of priority, beginning with the value which he gives the highest priority.

AN INVENTORY OF LIFE GOALS

The inventory of life goals is described to the client as an experience which offers him an opportunity for exploring and clarifying his life goals. Then the client is given a blank sheet of paper and asked to write the following at the top of the sheet: "These Are My Life Goals."

Then the client is asked to list his life goals. When he has completed the list of his goals, he is asked to place the list of basic values and the list of life goals side by side and examine them in the light of the following questions: (1) Are your values related to your life goals and vice versa?; or (2) Is what is of importance and worth to you related to what you wish to accomplish in your life?

The client may then be told that if he desires, he may write out his conclusions, including any changes he may feel are necessary.

If the client undertakes a systematic and planned clarification of his life goals and explores the relationships of these life goals to his basic values, this can lead to self-actualization by bringing basic values and life goals into closer harmony. The process of formulating a definite yet flexible set of life goals contributes to a feeling of self-confidence and inner freedom. The experience with the inventory of life goals can also help the client to achieve increased personal authenticity and add new dimensions to the search for personal identity.

THE ACHIEVEMENT IMAGERY EXPERIENCE

This technique was developed by Gibbons (1972) and is used for the mental realization of each goal listed by the client.

With the client in hypnosis, proceed with the following:

"I am going to count from one to five, and by the time I get to five, you will be mentally transported into the future, living and experiencing that attainment of [name the goal]. You will be able to hear my voice and respond to questions, and I will return you to the present time in a few minutes; but until I do so, the future event will be completely real to you as you experience it now . . . Going forward in time now. One . . . two . . . Going all the way forward to the attainment of [name the goal] . . . three . . . four . . . Almost there . . . five. Now you are in the future, feeling and experiencing the achievement of all you have hoped for in regard to [name the goal] . . . Live the attainment of this goal now, and experience all of the satisfaction and all of the feelings of achievement, and all of the happiness, pride, and joy that go with it . . . The perception and the feelings are becoming clearer and sharper now, and more distinct and more intense . . . As though it were the fulfillment of your very existence." [Gibbons, 1972, p. 11 and 12]

In hypnoanalysis, this phase is concerned with synthesis in addition to reeducation, because it is concerned with integration of the personality.

Before there can be true freedom in personality, there must be unity. The hypnosynthesis phase in hypnoanalysis includes interpretation, which relates the primitive infantile emotions to all later similar situations. Before therapy, these situations had been dealt with by repression and other defense mechanisms. This phase also includes the technique of the specific ideal model and an exercise in disidentification.

TECHNIQUE OF THE SPECIFIC IDEAL MODEL

The purpose of the technique of the specific ideal model is to utilize the plastic, creative and dynamic power of images, in particular visual images, within the client to develop a model of what he can become.

In utilizing this technique, it is essential that the client discard unrealistic and unworthy self-models. This should have been accomplished during the analytic phase.

The stages in the development of the specific ideal model are: first the idea, which, if seen as desirable, becomes an ideal; and then the form and function, which emerge when the ideal is ardently sought.

The technique of the specific ideal model is presented to the client as simply as possible. The following may be used as the first step in the technique: "See yourself now as you want to be, free from emotional disorder, free from pain, free from resentments. Picture the health, happiness and success which should be yours. Visualize yourself as the person you can become."

Frequently the building of the model is a collaboration in which the hypnotherapist tentatively presents the outline of the model and asks if it is acceptable or suggests to the client that he modify it, and especially that he complete it more concretely. The hypnotherapist then gives his approval and the client begins in the same session to build a model with the active help of the hypnotherapist, who assures the client that he too is building the same model with and for him.

The technique is carried out with the client in hypnosis. Emphasis is placed on the vividness and intensity of the visual evocation, not on its prolongation. The goal is a vivid, brief, repeated evocation; it is useful for the client to repeat it often.

The specific ideal model should be a well-defined and attainable model. The model should represent the next and most urgent step— that of focusing on a single specified quality or small group of qualities which the client most needs in order to proceed with his synthesis. He is asked to visualize himself in possession of that particular quality, and he is taught to see himself in a definite situation in which he puts into action the needed quality.

An autodrama in hypnosis can be developed in which the client sees himself in action playing several different roles. It can be suggested to the client that he visualize a scene fitting for each role, i.e., a scene in which he plays successfully and satisfactorily the role of son, husband, father, professional person, etc. By visualizing himself playing a particular role successfully, the client brings into action qualities which up to that time had not been sufficiently developed.

The hypnotherapist should encourage the client to relive the role in imagination and then seek to play it in reality. He should also be told not to care so much about the results, but rather to do the experiment in a detached manner. It should be stressed that the client always focus his greatest interest on the experiment itself and not on the practical results. This point can be a great help.

The exercises in disidentification and self-identification are focused on the control of the various elements of the personality. This is based on a fundamental psychological principle, which was formulated as follows by Gerard (1964):

"We are dominated by everything with which our self becomes identified. We can dominate and control everything from which we disidentify ourselves." Gerard continues: "The question becomes then to what extent can we identify ourselves with the true self and disidentify ourselves from the non-self."

For example, every time we identify ourselves with failure, we become more and more dominated by failure. The basic exercise of disidentification from the non-self and identification with the self is extremely important for synthesis. It is important to become aware that I have a body, but I am not my body. Sometimes I feel depressed, sometimes elated, sometimes loving. The moods change and are all passing, but I am not my feelings. I think, but I am not my thoughts. Then who am I? I am a self, a point of pure self-awareness. The next stage is the realization of one's true self, the discovery of this unifying center. The next step is the formation or reconstruction of personality around this unifying center.

THE EXERCISE IN DISIDENTIFICATION

The hypnotized client is told to repeat the following:

"I have a body but I am not my body. My body may find itself in different conditions of health or sickness; it may be rested or tired, but that has nothing to do with my self, my real 'I'. My body is my precious instrument of experience and of action in the outer world, but it is only an instrument. I treat it well; I seek to keep it in good health, but it is not myself. I have a body, but I am not my body.

"I have emotions, but I am not my emotions. These emotions are countless, contradictory, changing, and yet I know that I always remain I, myself, in times of hope or of despair, in joy or in pain, in a state of irritation or of calm. Since I can observe, understand and judge my emotions, and then increasingly dominate, direct and utilize them, it is evident that they are not myself. I have emotions, but I am not my emotions.

"I have desires, but I am not my desires, aroused by drives, physical and emotional, and by outer influences. Desires too are changeable and contradictory, with alternations of attraction and repulsion. I have desires but they are not myself.

"I have an intellect, but I am not my intellect. It is more or less developed and active; it is undisciplined but teachable; it is an organ of knowledge in regard to the outer world as well as the inner; but it is not myself. I have an intellect, but I am not my intellect." [Assagioli, 1971:118]

EXERCISE IN SELF-IDENTIFICATION

After the client successively disidentifies himself from his body ("I am not my body"), his emotions ("I am not my emotions"), his desires ("I am not my desires"), and his intellect ("I am not my intellect"), he proceeds to identify the "I" that remains, as a center of will. The following meditation is designed to get the client to experience his "I-ness" fully:

"What am I then? What remains after discarding from my self-identity the physical, emotional and mental contents of my personality, of my ego? It is the essence of myself—a center of pure self-consciousness and self-realization. It is the permanent factor in the ever-varying flow of my personal life. It is that which gives me the sense of being, of permanence, of inner security. I recognize and I affirm myself as a center of pure self-consciousness. I realize that this center not only has a static self-awareness but also a dynamic power; it is capable of observing, mastering, directing and using all the psychological processes and the physical body. I am a center of awareness and of power." [Assagioli, 1971, p. 19, 119]

Part Six

Hypnosis in Treatment

Chapter 21.

Accidental Autohypnosis: A Hypnocybernetic Approach to Emotional Disorders

The cause of an emotional disorder may be attributed to one specific factor or to a combination of factors. It is the contention of this author and others that most emotional disorders are caused by one or more of the following factors:

(1) conflict—wish to do something that taboos of society or conscience prevent;

(2) motivations—purposes the symptom may serve;

(3) identification;

(4) organ language—when the subconscious mind translates an idea into an actual physical condition, i.e., "that's a pain in the neck.";

(5) masochism—guilt is a frequent accompaniment to emotional disorders, along with its corollary, self-punishment;

(6) role of past experiences—we are to a great extent the product of the conditionings of our past experiences; and

(7) suggestion.

This chapter will deal with the seventh causative factor, suggestion, and its place in the formation of emotional disorders. Although it is by no means the only possible causal factor in emotional disorders, it is a most important one and one that has been largely ignored in the professional literature dealing with psychodiagnosis and psychotherapeutic treatment.

When a person is in the grip of an emotion, the subconscious mind takes over. Just as in hypnosis, there is no loss of consciousness and the person may unknowingly slip into a trance; just as in hypnosis, he becomes extremely suggestible. A remark may be made or the person may have a thought that is accepted or carried out by the subconscious mind as if it were a posthypnotic suggestion. Under intense emotion, the subconscious mind seems to automatically register a statement as though a tape recording is being made. With reinforcement through association (the same as posthypnotic suggestion) the idea will be carried out compulsively.

Hypnocybernetic, as used in the subtitle of this chapter, refers to the principles of cybernetics as applied to the human brain in conjunction with a decrease in organized brain activity. This decrease is due to a concentration of the mind that in turn is the result of an incident or idea of sufficient emotional importance.

Dr. Platonov (1959), a disciple of Pavlov, defined hypnosis as a decrease in organized cortical activity. The hypnotic state, therefore, is the same state that exists during an intense emotion; namely, a decreased organized brain activity.

Since the mental state produced by emotion is essentially the same as that following hypnotic induction, it may be termed "Accidental Autohypnosis."

Reflexes are present at birth and others may be acquired by repetition. It is possible, however, for a reflex to be acquired without repetition or conditioning. This can occur in the presence of emotion or during the state we refer to as hypnosis. Hypnosis and a strong emotional state are both mental states in which words act as signals and produce new reflexes without repetition.

A posthypnotic suggestion is the same as a conditioned reflex, but the signal is given at some time in the future. For example: "When you sit down to take the examination, you will feel calm, and your mind will be alert."

The acquiring of a reflex without repetition in the presence of emotion can be illustrated by the phenomenon of examination panic, as in the case of a student who is to take a test but is not completely prepared. When the student receives a copy of the test, he realizes that he doesn't know the answers to several of the questions on the first page and immediately feels that he is going to fail. Fear is the response and recall is impossible. As a result, he fails the exam. He is prepared for the next test, but when the exam questions are handed out, the emotion of fear returns; recall is in turn suppressed and he performs poorly.

In the above example, a situation was presented where it was essential to initiate conditioned reflexes necessary for recall. The response was fear. Fear caused such a decrease in organized brain activity that recall was impossible.

When emotion is present, it isn't necessary for an experience to be repeated in order for a reflex to develop. The stronger the emotion, the more readily new reflexes can be established and the more permanent they will become. During emotion, signals received can program the human computer (the brain). By this servomechanism, symptoms are able to continue long after the original cause has disappeared.

It has been scientifically proven that neurotic symptoms can be experimentally produced in normal subjects. Dr. A. R. Luria (1932), a Russian psychologist, described numerous experiments in which an artificial neurosis was produced by hypnosis. Self-hypnosis explains many of the extraordinary feats of yogis and fakirs.

It is realized today that all hypnosis is self-hypnosis; the subject must take the suggestion given to him by the hypnotic operator and give it to himself before hypnosis is accomplished. It is also known that a posthypnotic suggestion can be reinforced indefinitely through self-hypnosis. What is not usually realized is that self-hypnosis may occur accidentally and without the person's awareness.

According to Dr. S. J. Van Pelt (1956), President of the British Society of Medical Hypnotists, "If the mind is concentrated as the result of any incident or idea of sufficient emotional importance, then it is a condition of hypnosis. Any idea which is then introduced will act in the same way as a hypnotic command." [p. 30] When the individual finds himself experiencing an unpleasant feeling or emotion, he worries about it. The worry in turn creates more symptoms and sets up a vicious circle. Unpleasant bodily symptoms develop as a result of the effects of fear on the nervous system. The individual worries so much about the unpleasant symptoms that he forgets what first upset him.

Dr. Van Pelt was the first to point out that emotional disorders can be due to self-hypnosis. Indeed, Van Pelt believes that most emotional disorders, including the psychoses, are due to a form of self-hypnosis. Van Pelt (1958) gives the following illustration:

> Consider, for instance, a case of hysterical blindness. A soldier may be cut over the eyes by a shell splinter. The blood runs into his eyes so that he can't see. His mind is in a highly emotional state and we know that the emotion sensitizes the mind to hypnosis. The explosion has driven all thoughts out of his head except the one dominant thought which flashes through his mind: "My eyes, I can't see. I'm blind." In many cases he will be blind. In other words, he has induced blindness by self-hypnosis, just as a hypnotist could induce blindness in a susceptible person. He will remain blind until dehypnotized by some process, either a shock of sufficient magnitude or a hypnotist. [p. 15]

It was because of Van Pelt's ample proof of widespread accidental autohypnosis that stage hypnotism was banned in Great Britain (Van Pelt, 1961).

In another article, Dr. William J. Bryan (1961) stated:

> One of the basic principles of medical hypnosis proved by modern medical research is the fact that when an individual accepts an idea on an emotional and subconscious level, he alters his behavior pattern so that it conforms with the idea that he has accepted. Hence, if a patient is told that his left arm is paralyzed and he accepts this suggestion under hypnosis, he will act accordingly, living under this posthypnotic suggestion until it is removed. This is true whether the suggestion was introduced purposefully or accidentally. [p. 10]

In the practice of hypnoanalysis, I have encountered numerous individuals who have accidentally hypnotized themselves (through uncritical acceptance of a suggestion under intense emotion) into a false belief about themselves. These persons have been hypnotized by such false beliefs as "I am stupid," "I am unattractive," etc. With such self-definitions and self-conceptions, they have to fail in order to be true to their self-concept. Much of my time during hypnoanalytic sessions is spent in helping patients change their negative self-concepts by removing negative suggestions which were implanted when the patient was in a highly emotional state. It would be true to say that I dehypnotize these individuals, in the sense that they are helped to discover their true selves, which have been prevented from becoming a reality because they have accidentally hypnotized themselves into a negative, and therefore false, self-concept.

There is a rapidly expanding volume of medical literature confirming that a patient can hear while under chemical anesthesia. When a patient is under the influence of a general, chemical anesthetic, he may be considered to be in a state of parahypnosis. The term *parahypnosis* was coined by Van Dyke (1967) in his discussion of this condition which is still largely unknown by surgeons, anesthesiologists and nurses. In this state of parahypnosis, the patient is surgically insensitive to pain and is apparently unconscious, but he is able to hear voices and sounds. In parahypnosis, the patient is in a state of hypersuggestibility in which the brain centers primarily involved in critical evaluation are eliminated. This allows suggestions received by the patient to reach the deepest subconscious areas of the mind. Because the mind is concentrated by emotion and the situation in which the patient finds himself (surgery) is generally associated with a highly emotional state, suggestions given while the patient is in this state carry with them all the power of posthypnotic suggestions.

Cases have been reported of adverse effects of accidental autohypnosis induced while in church. Drs. Bryan and Millikin (1962) have reported two such cases. Dr. Bryan stated in his *Religious Aspects of Hypnosis* (1962) that hypnotic techniques in the utilization of a state of concentration in order to eliminate the stresses of the material world are more or less common in all religions. In discussing the many elements of hypnosis in religion, Bryan stated:

> The chanting, testimonials, the flickering candles and the cross as a fixation point for our vision; the relaxation of the rest of our body; the bowing of our heads in supplication; the silence in the Friend's meeting; Kavanah in Jewish mysticism; the preparation for prayer; the rotation of the body in the synagogue, and the effect of prayer on those who offer it, are all examples of hypnotic techniques which have been accepted as part of our own religious experience. [p. 25]

The mind is fixated and therefore highly suggestible in a church setting, and because hypnotic elements are used extensively during most church services, it may be said that many members of the congregation are in a state of hypnosis at least some of the time during the church service. The two cases cited above by Drs. Bryan and Millikin both involved the uncritical acceptance of the suggestion *fear of death*. In both cases, the ministers preached only on the negative aspect of death. The individuals, being in a state of hypnosis at the time, uncritically accepted the negative suggestions and developed emotional disorders as a result. It is important, therefore, that ministers, when speaking on the subject of death give greater emphasis to the theme of eternal life and avoid concentrating the sermon on death. It would also be good for doctors to be aware of the fact that patients who exhibit an undue preoccupation with or fear of death may have been influenced adversely during a period of accidental autohypnosis while in church.

Another example of accidental autohypnosis is the Walking Zombie Syndrome described by Dr. Bryan (1961). This is a condition in which the patient has accepted as fact, in his subconscious mind, the idea that he is already dead. This syndrome is identified and characterized by case histories containing statements such as "I have no vitality or life," and " I am very depressed and feel dead all the time." The incidence of this syndrome, according to Dr. Bryan, is very widespread. The correct treatment of the condition involves uncovering the Initial Sensitizing Event in which the patient accepted the suggestion that he was dead, as well as uncovering the Symptom Producing Event and subsequent Intensifying Events that increased the severity of the symptoms. A number of areas of the patient's history should be searched carefully in order to uncover these events. These include all early acute infectious diseases, accidents, injuries, operations, war experiences, and any deaths of close friends and members of the immediate family with whom the patient might have identified. Dr. Bryan presented nine cases that illustrate the numerous varieties of the presenting complaints, such as alcoholism, impotence, insomnia, depression, etc. In each case, the underlying cause was the acceptance of death as a reality by the patient's subconscious mind.

Dr. Bryan has described another syndrome that is the result of accidental autohypnosis, the Ponce de Leon Syndrome (1964). The victim of the Ponce de Leon Syndrome has accepted subconscious hypnotic suggestions that he can limit the aging process and that he is unable to grow older than a particular chronological age, resulting in subconscious fears of aging or of some danger that might occur as he grows older. The patient exhibits symptoms of behavior characteristic of the particular chronological age at which he is subconsciously fixated and is unable to compete effectively with other persons of his own chronological age. The symptoms most frequently include the inability to adopt any adult behavior or adult behavior in a particular area. Once the underlying fear of aging and the subconscious hypnotic suggestions that the patient had previously accepted are removed, the patient is then free to enjoy a normal aging process; in most cases, he will rapidly catch up to his actual chronological age level.

In summary, the hypnocybernetic theory of psychopathology provides us with a revolutionary theory of emotional disorders and how to treat them. It has been proven that symptoms identical with any emotional disorder can be experimentally produced in normal subjects. Furthermore, it has been shown that it is possible for a reflex to be acquired without repetition or conditioning, either in the presence of emotion or in hypnosis. Two syndromes, the Walking Zombie Syndrome and the Ponce de Leon Syndrome, which are due to accidental autohypnosis, have been presented, as well as the adverse effects of accidental autohypnosis induced while in church and while under chemical anesthesia.

Chapter 22.

The Treatment of Psychoneurotic Disorders by Hypnotherapy

The psychoneurotic disorders are among the most common of all forms of emotional disorder. Although the symptoms range from mild to disabling, the psychoneurotic person seldom needs to be institutionalized. Many of these cases respond favorably to hypnotherapeutic treatment.

The hypnotherapeutic treatment of the following psychoneurotic disorders will be discussed: anxiety reactions, hysterical conversion reactions, phobic reactions (anxiety hysteria), obsessive-compulsive reactions, and anxiety depression (reactive).

ANXIETY REACTIONS

Anxiety reactions occur when the total infantile experience of loss of life or of personal being itself is no longer able to be repressed, but is present within consciousness. The failure of repression permits both somatic and psychic elements of dread to emerge into consciousness. The symptoms are nonspecific and do not offer clues as to etiology. However, the precipitating factors and the setting in which attacks occur, especially the first attack, usually give clues to the underlying cause.

Anxiety can be manifested either as somatic or mental symptoms. The somatic symptoms can be diffusely spread throughout several body systems or chiefly limited to one system. The mental symptoms are subjective and may be manifested by difficulty in concentration, uneasiness, apprehension or fear of impending disaster.

In treating an anxiety reaction, it is almost mandatory to determine the underlying cause. Being brought to awareness of what is going on in his subconscious gives a person the best chance of overcoming his anxiety. During the analytic phase of treatment, an attempt is made to discover the sources of anxiety, their meaning and their historical origin. The duration of the treatment will depend upon the rigidity of personality and the extent to which the neurosis has been structuralized. The person must be shown how his present-day attitudes are distorted by anxieties rooted in past misconceptions and subconscious conflict; a reintegration to life and to people must be effected in the light of his new understanding.

It may not be possible to obtain an adequate history at the outset of treatment from a person in an acute state of anxiety. In such a case it would be best to commence with the induction of hypnosis. The history can then be elicited after the anxiety has diminished.

Hysterical Conversion Reactions

There is nothing essentially medical or organic about the simulated diseases of the hysterical conversion reaction. There may be little more at the base of the conversion reaction than the fact that in infancy, the quality of the mother's care was only satisfactory during periods of illness and that only cries of distress could bring the absent mother within sight of the infant. Both somatic and psychic elements are converted, within the subconscious, into a pseudodisease requiring attention. That is, the anxiety arising out of the conflicting situation is converted into somatic symptoms in parts of the body innervated by the sensorimotor system.

The somatic symptoms can vary widely. They frequently simulate organic disease and represent the person's idea of the disease process. Conversion reactions chiefly involve organs which are in contact with the external world. The distribution of symptoms is unphysiological and nonanatomical. The somatic symptoms can be manifested in diverse ways, such as paralysis, blindness, deafness or convulsive states.

The outstanding mental symptom is the person's indifference to his illness. Although he obviously has disabling symptoms, he appears unconcerned and shows no anxiety.

The choice of symptom may be determined by:

(1) the experience of the organ in relation to the conflict (i.e., paralysis of a hand with which the person has struck or has wished to strike someone in anger);

(2) suitability of the organ to express the conflict symbolically (i.e., paralysis of the legs as a defense against action); and

(3) events tending to focus the conflict in a specific area (i.e., a tonsillectomy may be the precursor to aphonia—the inability to utter sounds—as an expression of an underlying conflict operating at the time of surgery).

Persons with a proneness to hysterical personality may first draw attention to the onset of organic illness by hysterical conversion reactions. That is why it is important that a diagnosis be made by a physician in all cases.

A strong secondary gain element is almost always operative after the formation of a conversion reaction. The ego exploits the symptom to further the person's security pursuits. A patient may gain sympathy, financial compensation, and freedom from undesirable duties through the illness. This factor must always be kept in mind in therapy. Incentives to get well must be created to offset the benefits of continuing symptoms. The treatment of conversion reaction is dependent upon the motivation of the person and the role the existing symptoms play in his life adaptational scheme.

Such symptoms as hysterical paralysis, aphonia, visual disorders of a hysterical nature, hysterical anesthesias and hysterical contractures may be removed in relatively few sessions by means of hypnotic suggestion with a strong authoritarian approach. However, one must not overestimate the permanency of cure, since the original motivations that caused the symptoms to manifest themselves are not altered in the least, and a relapse is always possible. Consequently, the person should be encouraged to pursue further therapy of a hypnoanalytic type for an explanation of the nature of his symptom and its source in unconscious conflict.

The treatment of hysterical conversion reactions through hypnotic symptom removal is least successful where the symptom serves the purpose of providing intense substitute gratification for sexual and hostile impulses. Here hypnoanalysis will be useful.

PHOBIC REACTIONS (ANXIETY HYSTERIA)

Phobic reactions are disorders of movement in relation to significant people or things. The hysterical reaction is based on separation-anxiety; as a disorder of movement, it is an anxious inability to move away from people. The schizoid personality disorder is basically a commitment-anxiety. If people come close to the schizoid person, he is compelled to move away in order to remain at a safe distance. As a phobic disorder of movement, this may be termed an inability to move toward people. The depressive personality is basically an aggression-anxiety. Expressed as a phobic disorder of movement, it is an inability to move against people.

The term *phobic reaction* is most commonly associated with the hysterical position. That is why Freud used the term *anxiety hysteria.* By means of a phobia, the fixated separation-panic is kept out of consciousness by projecting it upon unconsciously determined external situations. Commonly, the phobia is a symbolic representation of the underlying impulse or desire. Some phobias represent fear of punishment for the underlying unacceptable desire.

Aside from the phobia itself, the other symptoms are chiefly concerned with ways of avoiding the feared object or situation. The phobic person has focalized his anxiety, and as long as he can avoid the focalized object, he remains relatively comfortable and free of anxiety. If confronted with the phobic object or situation, the person develops anxiety. He recognizes the unreasonableness of the phobia, but is unable to control his behavior.

The main determinants of phobic reactions will be found to be involved with unsatisfactory interpersonal relationships in the days or weeks preceding the phobic attack; the primitive origin of many phobic reactions can be traced to the birth experience itself.

A careful history taking is in itself a valuable therapeutic activity. It concentrates the person's attention on his interpersonal relationships where the present difficulty lies. As Sullivan (1953) stated: "A much more practical psychotherapy seems to be possible when one seeks to find the basic vulnerabilities to anxiety in interpersonal relations, rather than to deal with symptoms called out by anxiety or to avoid anxiety." When this has been satisfactorily clarified, we discover what presently lies behind the phobic symptom.

It is valuable to explain to persons suffering from phobic reactions the nature and development of infantile personality. If they can familiarize themselves with the quality of anxiety that lies behind the phobic reaction, they are draining the fear that has been concentrated in the phobic object.

It is also desirable to encounter the primitive anxiety and to experience it fully in consciousness and evacuate it from the subconscious. If this can be done, then the primal determinant of the phobia has ceased to exist. There is then little difficulty in overcoming the reluctance to face the feared object.

Where the phobic reaction is the product of a character pattern that originated early in life, it will be necessary to produce a reorganization of the personality through hypnoanalysis. Where the phobic reaction is not indicative of an underlying conflict and the individual has a relatively stable personality with no neurotic character structure, then direct hypnotherapy will be effective.

Obsessive-Compulsive Reactions

The obsessive-compulsive reaction is characterized by obsessions and/or compulsions. Obsessions are recurring ideas or impulses that remain in consciousness despite their irrationality. Common themes are violence, sexuality, religion, and obscenities. Compulsions are recurring acts that develop as a means of relieving obsessions or fears. Common themes expressed in the compulsive acts are contamination and self-mutilation. Because the person is often embarrassed about his compulsions and rituals, he often goes to great lengths to disguise them from others. If the compulsions become more severe or chronic, his ability to hide the acts becomes progressively less successful.

This reaction is dynamically more complicated than any of the other psychoneurotic reactions. Repression is unsuccessful (or only partially successful), and the person resorts to other defense mechanisms to reinforce the repression. These subsequent defenses are most often isolation and reaction formation; however, every defense mechanism may be used in the severe cases of obsessive-compulsive reactions.

Isolation is characterized by the interposition of a blank pause after a highly unpleasant or personally significant experience. Reaction formation is manifested in irrational and sometimes excessive action in the opposite direction to an impulse or desire which is being repressed.

The obsessive-compulsive person is usually intelligent, and often is rigid, restricted, orderly, meticulous, conscientious and dependable. Unlike the person who has a hysterical conversion reaction, the obsessive-compulsive person is uncomfortable and is dealing more actively with his conflict.

The dynamics of obsessive-compulsive reactions are closely related to the schizoid position; therefore, the problem of treatment is fundamentally the same.

The treatment of obsessive-compulsive reactions must take into account the person's dependency, the profoundly hostile impulses he has toward people, his need for detachment, the tendency to isolate intellect from feeling, and the magical frame of reference in which his ideas operate. Among the most important tasks to be achieved are demonstrating to the client that his symptoms have a definite cause and that they stem from no magical source; that aggression is a normal impulse originating in hostile attitudes; that he can express a certain amount of hostility without destroying other people or injuring himself; that he can relate to a person without needing to make himself dependent or compliant.

Obsessive-compulsive reactions generally do not respond to an analytic approach as well as do other psychoneurotic syndromes.

A directive reeducational approach that uses guidance and reassurance appears to be the best treatment approach. As soon as the client achieves as deep a state of hypnosis as can be brought about, he is given reassuring suggestions to the effect that he can get well, that others sicker than himself have been able to experience relief from their symptoms, and that, if he has the desire to recover, he will want to do what is essential in overcoming his difficulties.

One of the most important things he is to realize is that his symptoms are not the product of supernatural forces, but rather follow scientific laws of cause and effect. The reasons he suffers will become known to him as he begins to connect events in his environment with how he feels. Accepting this explanation on faith is not enough. It is essential to point out to the client how, when he gets involved in specific environmental difficulties, his symptoms become exacerbated.

An explanation of the dynamics of his disorder may be given to the client. This approach, utilizing concepts that he is intellectually capable of comprehending, gives him a far more reasonable explanation for his illness than the confused situation that he has customarily imagined to exist. Once he has begun to divest his thinking of its magical associations, he will be able to absorb deeper insights and to use them in the direction of change.

A persuasive technique may also be employed in hypnosis. The client is told that were he actually going to carry his obsessive thoughts into action, he would do so without tormenting himself. The chances are that he will not perpetrate any of the wicked deeds of which he is so frightened.

One of the tendencies of the obsessive-compulsive person is an impulse to keep tormenting himself with his fears and anxieties. It should be pointed out to the client while in hypnosis that occupying his mind with frightening ideas stirs up tension and physical symptoms.

The client is told that suggestions will be given him to switch the type of thinking that preoccupies him. What is necessary is that the obsessive-compulsive person begin to direct thoughts away from concern with his obsessions to some other group of thoughts, no matter what they may be. This could be some activity or hobby, or some period in life when his happiness was greatest.

ANXIETY DEPRESSION (REACTIVE)

The depression in these cases is usually set off by an external event, such as loss of a loved one. Insofar as the environmental deprivation is causative, we can say that the depression is exogenous or reactive. Persons suffering from reactive depression show evidence that they have a great deal of repressed mental pain—deducible by the number of defensive reaction patterns deriving from traumatic levels of separation anxiety into which they have been driven (i.e., hysterical, schizoid, phobic, obsessional).

Agitation and overt anxiety are usually present. Guilt feelings and self-accusations are often mixed with feelings of resentment. These persons often demand help and are accessible to hypnotherapy.

Behind reactive depression is rage, and behind rage, privation and separation-anxiety. Privation refers to a diminishing capacity to be-in-relatedness with the source person, thus increasing separation-anxiety.

There are major goals in the treatment of the depressed person. First, it is of great importance to foster the awareness of the unacceptable hostility that exists. Second, these intense emotions must be made acceptable, so that the person can learn to express them without activating massive guilt feelings. Third, the faulty parental introjects must be replaced with values that are both realistic and attainable.

The attainment of a complete history serves a double purpose. It not only gives the hypnotherapist a greater understanding of the dynamics of the disorder, but also aids considerably in the establishment of rapport.

Although it is unlikely that difficulties would arise in the establishment of rapport with the depressed person, hypnosis is of definite value in fostering its rapid development.

When hypnotic rapport has been established, treatment should gradually be directed toward the fostering of insight into the profound feelings of resentment that have been so deeply repressed. This can be approached most effectively through inducing the person to recall the many frustrations in his life. As situation after situation is remembered, the depressed client very gradually becomes aware of the justification for some of the anger on his part.

The fostering of insight is one of the most valuable contributions of hypnosis to the therapeutic process. The length of treatment can be dramatically reduced through the effective employment of unconscious recall. It should be stressed, however, that any uncovering carried out during hypnosis should be followed by the instructions: "When the hypnotic state is lifted, you will recall only those things that you wish to remember." This not only insures the client's progression at his own pace, but enables the hypnotherapist to gauge effectively which materials can be worked through at a conscious level and which areas should be continued under hypnosis.

In this fashion, the depressed client gradually becomes cognizant of his profound feelings of resentment toward those people to whom he has never dared express anger. Insight, however, is not sufficient to ameliorate the problem. The depressed person must learn to accept and express these feelings. It is through the introjective process that this takes place.

New learning can most effectively be instilled in the client through a systematic emphasis on the normality, appropriateness, and the healthiness of justified expressions of anger. Each time the depressive person responds in this manner, reward in the form of approval must be given. When a suppressive or repressive response is made, disapproval should be given. This, however, must not imply rejection. To strengthen further the new learning, the therapist himself must be able to demonstrate to the depressed person that he too can express anger when the situation justifies it.

With the continued expression of these once-taboo feelings, the client gradually gains the impression that hostility is not as evil as he had been taught, certainly not, if the hypnotherapist, the omnipotent good parent figure, can express this affect. As this emotion becomes more acceptable, the depressed person allows himself freer expression. The reinforcement continues until the response is strengthened to the point where it can be directed at the original source of the frustration. When this can be accomplished without stirring up intensive guilt feelings, the depressive defense is no longer required.

The awareness, acceptance and expression of these hostile emotions creates intensive guilt which the client cannot bear. Each time he approaches this tension-provoking feeling, he tends to retreat. The immediate tension reduction is sufficiently rewarding to cause this withdrawal to persist. Although the later reward of freedom from guilt, anxiety, and depression would be much greater, the immediate pain reduction, because of its immediacy, is of greater reward value.

Suggestions should be continually given that anger is a normal and appropriate emotion that is evoked in certain situations. When frustration is present, anger should be expressed in a logical and realistic fashion. The repeated employment of posthypnotic suggestions has been demonstrated to be an effective means of altering long-standing attitudes.

Hypnosis can also be highly valuable in the creation of artificial frustrating situations, to which the client is directed to respond in an angry manner. As these reactions are rewarded, the response itself becomes sufficiently reinforced so that with continued conditioning, hostility will be spontaneously evoked in a real situation without provoking undue guilt.

Chapter 23.

The Treatment of Personality Disorders by Hypnotherapy

The term *personality disorder* is an unfortunate one since it has been used in a popular way to mean all personality disturbances, equating personality disorder with emotional disorder. The diagnostic category is quite broad, and it is complicated by the somewhat unrelated nature of the conditions included in it. Only three broad diagnostic categories will be discussed in this chapter: the schizoid personality, the psychopathic personality, and sexual deviations. While the sexual deviations were grouped under the heading of psychopathic personality in the past, the current diagnostic classification considers the sexual deviate apart from the psychopathic or antisocial type of personality disorder. "Such a separation in classification is important because, while many sexually deviant acts are the result of an antisocial personality, many others grow out of personality dynamics of a quite different kind." (Kisker, 1964). [p. 233]

THE SCHIZOID PERSONALITY

The schizoid personality is characterized by the following: an enduring pattern of behavior manifesting avoidance of close relationships with others; the inability to express hostility and aggressive feelings directly; autistic thinking, i.e., thinking that is controlled by the wishes of the individual at the expense of the information actually available from the external world; and a seclusive, withdrawn, introverted personality.

The presence of schizoid components in the personality are indicative of a person who always has a strong death wish. Personal being by relatedness to a source person has been irreparably destroyed. The schizoid position is the exact opposite of the hysterical position. The hysterical position is characterized by separation-anxiety, whereas the schizoid position is characterized by nonseparation anxiety or commitment-anxiety.

The schizoid position refers to the existence, deeply repressed from consciousness, of the original traumatic experience of the splitting of the personality. The deepest split is associated with traumatic experiences in infancy. The schizoid position is synonymous with an experience of unbearable dread or of identification with nonbeing.

The essence of the schizoid position is despair. The dread and despair of the schizoid position has at its core a total loss of personal identity.

Guntrip has described the schizoid person as one who has

> very early in life encountered love-starvation. His personal needs have been repeatedly excited without being satisfied and he came to react to this intolerable state of affairs by getting, firstly, more and more hungry and needy, and developing a greedy, demanding, devouring attitude to all love-objects. Then he became afraid because his love, or need for love, had grown so exorbitant as to seem, and even be destructive. He became afraid to need and love, and withdrew mentally into a state of not having any needs and feelings. In the course of time, a definite character developed, marked by detachment, aloofness and coldness . . . If the schizoid personality begins to break down, it is usually into apathy, loss of interest, and a sense of futility, unreality and pointlessness in life. He may commit suicide with a calculated bored attitude of 'there's no point in going on living.' His needy libidinal ego is utterly crushed and imprisoned within, and all human warmth has gone . . . The schizoid is the complete introvert. [1957, pp. 101-103]

The schizoid person lives in a world made up of a depersonalized self and of depersonalized others. He is in flight from personalization and has assumed a position of self-sustaining isolation. He encounters feelings of despair when he tries to force himself back into commitment. The depersonalization of the schizoid person is actively sought and is often accompanied by a profound death wish. If the schizoid person does seek out help, then there still remains a part of the person that is actively protesting against depersonalization, and it is with this lifeseeking element that we must work.

The onset of the schizoid position is associated with feelings of nonbeing and the unreality of the self. The precipitating factor is a threat to the continuance of dependence upon personal sources which has led to the emergence into conscious awareness of an infantile experience of identification with nonbeing (depersonalization) that was so traumatic that it had to be split off from the acceptable self and repressed. There was buried alive a painful experience that said, "If my mother isn't real, I am not real and my world isn't real." Any circumstances that weaken repression in later life may lead to a failure of repression of infantile depersonalization experiences so that they emerge into conscious awareness. The indwelling human spirit is threatened by loss of reality and loss of selfhood.

The initial emphasis in treatment must be on the creation of a human relationship with the schizoid sufferer that has pleasure values for him. Only by this means will he relinquish the safety of detachment. The handling of treatment requires considerable tact. No matter how detached, the person is extremely sensitive to everything the therapist says or does. Avoidance of situations that evoke anxiety is essential.

Frequently during treatment, the schizoid person will react with detachment or withdrawal, or he may subject the therapist to a testing period, during which he is hostile. The testing period may be a trying one for the therapist, since it may continue for many months, during which the schizoid person constantly rejects the therapist. When he realizes that the therapist doesn't expect him to do certain things, he will begin to reevaluate him in a new light.

The beginning of a feeling of closeness may precipitate panic, and the schizoid person may try to run away from therapy or exhibit aggression toward the therapist. The ability to see the schizoid through this stage finally may succeed in breaking down his reserve and in establishing for the first time an identification with a person based upon unconditional acceptance.

Once a positive relationship has been established, it is necessary to use it in order to strengthen the ego of the schizoid person. Nothing must jeopardize the therapeutic relationship. The schizoid person's feelings and attitudes must be respected at all times. It is unnecessary and even undesirable to reinforce these attitudes by agreeing with them, but they should be accepted as something the person believes, even though there might be another explanation than the one he imagines. All probing for dynamic material should be avoided until the ego is sufficiently strong to cope with it.

Initially, the therapist would proceed with hypnoidal therapy, emphasizing relaxation, calmness and inner peace of mind and making judicious use of explanation and persuasion.

THE PSYCHOPATHIC PERSONALITY

Greenwald (1967) divides the psychopath into two broad categories. The first is the sociopath, the individual who is conforming to the norms of the environment in which he grew up. For example, he might have grown up in a neighborhood where antisocial behavior was so widespread that in order to be properly adjusted to his society, he developed into a deviant. The second category of psychopath is one who has grown up in a milieu that does not share such deviant norms. Greenwald refers to such a person as an individual psychopath or character neurotic.

Although psychopaths are usually described as lacking morality, this is not completely true, because they frequently have a moral code of their own. Another fallacy is that psychopaths are free of anxiety. If a workable relationship is established in therapy, then the anxiety becomes quite clear.

In order to develop a workable relationship with the psychopathic person, it is absolutely essential for the therapist to keep his morality to himself, at least in the initial stages of therapy.

The next problem in the treatment of the psychopath is that of fees. According to Greenwald, it does no good to set limits (i.e., "I'll give you two months and if you don't pay we will stop treatment"). What you have to do is to discuss payment of the fee continually.

The next problem in treating psychopaths is that of seduction. Psychopathic personalities practice many types of seductive behavior in their attempts to manipulate.

The central problem in the therapy of the psychopathic personality is the problem of control. The therapist must demand control within the therapy session if he expects the psychopathic person to gain control over himself outside of therapy. His major problem is that he didn't learn controls when he was young. Very explicit ground rules have to be established at the outset of therapy and continuously maintained. One good ground rule is to prohibit socializing with other clients outside of therapy. Another good rule for developing self-control is to prohibit smoking during therapy sessions.

After control has been established, the next step is to facilitate the verbal expression of the psychopathic person's hostility and, more important, what is hidden behind the hostility—in most cases enormous dependency needs.

Greenwald has used hypnosis in conjunction with relationship therapy in treating psychopathic persons and reports that the use of hypnosis in the therapy of the psychopath is often a shortcut to a workable relationship.

Dr. Robert Lindner wrote an entire book, *Rebel Without a Cause* (1944) on the treatment of a psychopathic personality with hypnoanalysis. In his summary chapter Lindner stated:

Through hypnoanalysis, we have been able to obtain meaningful insights into the psychogenesis of the criminal psychopathic state. For the first time, we have been privileged to penetrate beneath the armor which persons of such classification present to the world, and to view in all their sinister automaticity the operationism of the responsible mechanisms. With but little effort, we can reconstruct the peculiar constellation of events which formed the attitudes that influenced Harold's later behavior. We have observed the introjective process at work as it split off from the environment and absorbed all those singular and crucial events which later crystallized into habits of response and particular ways of viewing the setting against which subsequent behavior was enacted . . . The prepotency of hypnoanalysis could have been demonstrated with no greater forcefulness than it has been through its success with psychopathic personality, a condition which has resisted other investigative and therapeutic techniques. It is quite likely that the resistant nature of this disorder derives from the fact that it engulfs the whole personality, somewhat in the manner of a psychosis, from the very earliest age, and that one of its peculiar symptoms is an inability to come into rapport with anyone . . . In the case reviewed, the patient was "cured" in the sense of alteration of style of life, and imbued with a real ability to live with his particular ocular symptom. The alteration was based on what some psychologists call "insight," on a real understanding of the past and a reorientation of attitudes and aims. [pp. 317, 318 & 320]

In his discussion of the use of hypnosis in the treatment of the psychopathic personality, Wolberg (1948) stated:

> The treatment of the heterogeneous disorder which has been given the loose term "psychopathic personality" is facilitated to a marked degree by the employment of hypnosis. . . . Psychopaths are easily hypnotized with a proper technique . . . Direct advice in the hypnotic state is usually more acceptable to the patient than in the waking state, and suggestions may be couched in such terms as to convince the patient that he is actually wiser and happier for resisting certain activities which, on the basis of past experience, are bound to result disastrously. On the basis of a guidance relationship, the patient may be taught the wisdom of postponing immediate gratifications for those which, in the long run, will prove more lasting and wholesome. He is taught the prudence of tolerating frustration, and the need to feel a sense of responsibility and consideration for the rights of others. Not that these lessons will be accepted or acted on, but constant repetition sometimes helps the patient realize that it is to his best interests, in the long run, to observe social amenities and to exercise self control. [pp. 318, 320, 321]

If the psychopathic person is capable of achieving somnambulism with the eyes open, hypnotic play therapy can be very beneficial therapeutically. During hypnotic play therapy, the individual acts out his fantasies as well as anxiety-provoking real life situations.

Hypnotic play therapy is especially suited to the expression of subconscious aggression. It may be utilized both at adult and regressed age levels.

A wide variety of materials should be available before attempting to do play therapy. Among the most important materials are a set of dolls comprising a mother and father, a grandmother and grandfather, a boy and girl, a baby, and several dolls representing authority figures such as a policeman and a clergyman. Other materials are toy animals, a dollhouse and doll furniture, toy cars, airplanes, guns, soldiers, a rubber dagger, a nursing bottle, play dough, paper and crayons.

In play therapy, the client projects his feelings onto the play materials. Wolberg (1945) felt that the play therapy interview should be conducted in the third person, unless the client identifies himself with one of the dolls and appears to be cognizant of what is going on. A posthypnotic amnesia may be suggested by telling the client that he will gradually understand at a conscious level the significance of the play.

SEXUAL DEVIATIONS

Modern textbooks of hypnotherapy, if they deal with the treatment of sexual disorders at all, generally give scant and vague information. Furthermore, there is a paucity of articles in the professional literature pertaining to the treatment of the various sexual disorders by hypnotherapy. Obstinate sexual disorders of all types appear to be susceptible to hypnotherapy. To a great extent, this was known more than 80 years ago but appears to have been forgotten.

The sexual deviations should all be treated by hypnoanalysis, because in most cases they are manifestations of a deep-seated conflict. In all cases the hypnoanalysis should be followed by reeducation and in many cases by reconditioning. The following sexual deviations will be briefly discussed: transvestism, exhibitionism, pedophilia, voyeurism, fetishism, and homosexuality.

When treating the sexual deviate, it is always important to keep in mind that he didn't originally start out to seek gratification by abnormal means. In the early period of development, the deviate displayed normal sexual functioning, heterosexual experiences and phantasies, although there may have been intrapsychic conflicts present at an early age. This apparently normal sexual functioning may have lasted through puberty and even through adolescence. The basis on which to found the hypnotherapy is an investigation of when the turn to deviate sexual gratification occurred. Then the disorder is traced back to its roots, when conflicts about sexual objects first appeared, by means of age regression and other hypnoanalytic techniques, and the reasons for the distorted development are discovered.

The sexual deviation of the patient is an expression of his whole personality structure. His phantasy life has to be explored and exposed. This will help the patient to recognize and accept the fact that his way of seeking sexual gratification is a defense and a flight from his deepest desire, heterosexuality.

As every sexual deviation is mixed with different neurotic symptomatology, the therapeutic aim will also shift at times. In addition, the therapist must consider the possible changes that he feels the patient is capable of attaining. Attention, therefore, must constantly be paid to ego strength and to frustration tolerance.

Transvestism

This is a deviation in which sexual satisfaction is obtained by wearing the clothing of the opposite sex and by genital contact with such clothing. The transvestite often tends to feel and act like a member of the opposite sex.

Friedman (1959) summarized the psychoanalytical view of transvestism as follows:

> Here too, as in many other perversions, there is an attempt at reassurance against castration anxiety. This arises from the infantile belief that the woman has lost her penis as a result of castration; hence, the subject, too, might become a victim of castration. By donning female clothing and by continuing to receive sensations from the penis, the transvestite unconsciously identifies with a phallic woman whose penis is hidden by her clothing.

First of all, it should be determined what type of transvestite the individual is. Hirschfield (1944) believed there were ten types, including the following: the complete transvestite, the extreme transvestite, who wants to change his sex; the partial transvestite, who is content to wear the underclothing of the opposite sex; the periodic transvestite, who switches back and forth; the narcissistic transvestite, who is all absorbed with himself; the bisexual transvestite and the homosexual transvestite.

The transvestite should be treated in reconstructive hypnoanalysis, because he usually has a strong feminine role identification in addition to castration anxiety; a reconstruction of character structure is necessary. If the individual wants to change his sex, or if he is a narcissist, bisexual or homosexual, these should be considered as the primary symptoms and dealt with as such, the transvestism being only secondary.

After the transvestism has been traced to its origin and worked through at an emotional level during the analytic phase of treatment, reeducation of attitudes and deconditioning of the habit pattern are usually necessary. A form of aversive conditioning such as an electric shock associated with dressing in clothes of the opposite sex may be employed during the deconditioning phase of treatment.

EXHIBITIONISM

The exhibitionist obtains relief from sexual tension by exposing a part of his body, especially the genitals. The exhibitionist is basically shy and conscientious. His behavior is characterized by a claustrophobic anxiety, manifested by a feeling of insecurity in his own home. He is usually impotent and sexually prudish and is often riddled with deep feelings of guilt and the need to be punished. This is shown by his compulsion to return to the scene of his exhibitionistic acts until he is eventually reported and apprehended.

As Karpman (1954) stated, the exhibitionist

> depends for satisfaction on the reaction of the women to whom he exposes himself. His overwhelming need is to find an outlet for frustration set up by his forbidden goal, incest. He gains no real sexual pleasure; the act is a violent attempt to deny the buried incestuous drive, an unconscious choice of the lesser of two evils. He is a compulsive neurotic . . . rigid, isolated, sheltered, orderly, all for one purpose, protection . . . He is subservient to mother but inwardly rebels . . . He has never learned adult sexual conduct. The relief from tension is the same as other compulsives obtained from obsessive rites. [p. 370]

Exhibitionistic attacks may take place every day, once a week, once a month, or they may be limited to merely one episode. The onset of an attack is marked restlessness, anxiety, and apprehension. Physical symptoms are often headache, palpitation, perspiration, and a feeling of sexual excitement.

After exposure, the exhibitionist is usually filled with remorse and relief. The remorse comes from feelings of guilt, the relief because the act is one of sexual fulfillment. Usually, he resolves never to repeat the act, but because he acts compulsively, he is often unable to resist at a later date.

Fenichel (1945) stated,

> In exhibitionism, a denial of castration is attempted by a simple overcathexis of a partial instinct. Reassurance against castration can be obtained by an exhibitionistic man in the following way: he unconsciously says to his audience, "reassure me that I have a penis by reacting to the sight of it." Inner doubt impels the individual to call upon objects as witness. [p. 345]

Although hypnoanalysis is the preferred treatment for working through the obsessive-compulsive neurosis and the castration anxiety, hypnosuggestion will prove to be very beneficial in conjunction with the hypnoanalysis. Ritchie (1968) gave the following hypnotic suggestions, in a case of exhibitionism during the first and each of the following hypnotic sessions:

(1) You are a healthy normal male with a normal size penis . . .; (2) You do not have to be frightened by any woman, for no woman or anyone will ever cut off your penis; (3) When you begin to develop a tight, tense feeling in the pit of your stomach and lower chest, this feeling will be immediately relieved by putting your right hand in your pants pocket and letting the tip end of your fingers touch the side of your penis which will assure you that it is there and of normal size; and (4) When you awaken from these sessions you will feel totally at peace, utterly relaxed, and as if you had had four hours of complete restful sleep. [pp. 41, 42]

Constructive realistic phantasies (Levitsky, 1966) may be used effectively with the exhibitionist. The suggestion can be given that when he awakens he will have an overwhelming desire to exhibit himself to the hynotherapist with all of the symptoms of tension and whatever other symptoms he has always experienced whenever he exhibited himself. In addition, the conditioning technique of Ritchie (1968) is very effective. The patient is told that the desire to exhibit himself will increase for three seconds after he awakens, and then when he has reached the place where the feelings are becoming totally unbearable, he will put his right hand in his pocket and let his fingers just touch the side of his penis and this will be immediately relieved, and that it will be so dramatic that he will remember to do this whenever he has any tendency to exhibit himself.

PEDOPHILIA

Pedophilia, or child sexuality, refers to the use of an immature person as a sexual object, with the relationship based on either a homosexual or a heterosexual inclination. The pedophiliac is often frightened by adult sexuality. The child presents less of a threat and because of naivete often becomes a willing victim.

It is Dr. Bryan's contention that many child molesters are victims of the Ponce de Leon Syndrome (Bryan, 1964).

Many child molesting cases can easily be explained by the simple acceptance of a hypnotic suggestion to the effect that the patient is at an age level in which such behavior is acceptable. In personal communication with a number of judges who have tried such cases, many of them are astounded at the fact that the child molester frequently does not "molest" the child at all and that in many cases the children are not injured in any way but that the man is merely carrying out the same type of investigative behavior that he might have done at age six, seven, or eleven which would have been considered normal at that age but which because the man is 39, 52, or 70 is considered distinctly abnormal, or even criminal. The failure to understand the cause of such child molestation or such "childlike sexual behavior" has led to the incarceration of these individuals, when in reality they need hypnotic medical treatment . . . Many patients are arrested in their sexual development only at a specific age level . . . the cause in each case is that the subconscious mind of the individual has merely accepted a suggestion which if accepted would result in the arresting of some part of the individual's life at a particular age level. The individual is brainwashed in the Fountain of Youth. (A tragic bath indeed). [p. 36]

VOYEURISM

Voyeurism refers to the practice of men who derive erotic satisfaction in looking at either naked women or the sexual act performed by others. The observation of sexually arousing situations becomes a substitute for participation in such activities.

In discussing the psychodynamics of voyeurism, Kisker (1964) has stated that

In some cases, the voyeur is seeking reassurance. A common psychoanalytic interpretation is that such patients are preoccupied with scenes which have aroused castration anxiety. In other cases, there is an overt sexual pleasure experienced by means of identification with one of the persons when a sex act is witnessed. Another possible explanation is in terms of the forbidden nature of the act. [p. 236]

Hypnoanalysis is necessary to uncover the cause of the voyeurism as well as reconstructing the neurotic character structure into a mature, adult character structure. All aspects of an individual's life are interconnected. The sexually immature person, which every sexual deviate most certainly is, is also emotionally immature. After the meaning of the voyeurism has been determined and the Initial Sensitizing Event, Symptom Producing Event and Symptom Intensifying Events have been revivified and worked through at a conscious level, the patient still needs reeducation and hypnosuggestion for the reinforcement of healthy adult attitudes toward sex.

FETISHISM

In fetishism, the object of the sexual drive is either a part of the human body, such as hair, hands, feet, legs, breasts or buttocks, or an article of clothing, such as stockings, shoes, underwear or handkerchiefs. Fetishism occurs much more often among men than women.

In discussing fetishism, Kling (1965) explained true sexual fetishism as existing

> in the fact that the individual experiences a sexual emotion on seeing the object, in the absence of the person, and that he can obtain not only an erection by fondling or caressing the object but an orgasm as well. In short, the true fetishist finds in the object a substitute for all desire for sexual intercourse. [p. 246]

Behavior of this kind is often a conditioned response established during childhood. It may take the form of kissing and fondling an article of clothing or other items belonging to the person to whom the strong emotional attachment has been built up. There is a displacement of sexual excitement to an object that accidentally accompanied the first sexual experiences of the child.

After being trained to go as deep as possible in hypnosis, the client is instructed to recall every important impression or experience he has had with regard to sex and with regard to the object of the fetishism, beginning with the first incident. He is encouraged to relive each incident connected with the development of the fetishism and the sexual excitement connected with the object is removed through appropriate suggestions and reeducation. Since behavior of this kind has often developed into a conditioned response pattern, the analytic phase of treatment should be followed by a period of desensitization so that the patient becomes desensitized to the object of his fetishism and the habit pattern is broken.

As with transvestites, there has been some success with aversive conditioning in the treatment of fetishism. McGuire and Vallance (1964) reported the successful use of aversive conditioning with a 25-year-old postgraduate student who had been masturbating for ten years approximately three times a day to fantasies of himself dressed in blue jeans and a leather jacket, and to masochistic fantasies of being bound. After aversion therapy was explained to him, he was told to conjure up his usual fantasies and to give a signal by raising his hand when the image was clear. When he did so, the shock was administered. This was sufficient to dispel the fantasy. The patient reported that he found it increasingly difficult to conjure up the fantasy that was being treated. At later sessions he was unable to conjure up his usual fantasies. Photographs of people dressed in his fetishist clothing were used as stimuli, at first producing interest and excitement, but even this soon disappearing. From the day treatment started, he had never masturbated to his fantasies, and this remained true during the one year of follow-up.

HOMOSEXUALITY

One of the most common forms of sexual deviation is homosexuality. A homosexual is one whose sexual urges are directed principally or exclusively toward persons of his own sex.

There are conflicting theories as to the etiology of homosexuality. Most psychoanalysts believe that homosexuality is a case of arrested sexual development and represents hidden but incapacitating fears of the opposite sex.

Dr. Albert Ellis (1965) and others have pointed out that many individuals engaging in homosexual acts may have become fixed at a particular developmental level and are unable to go on, either because of fear or some other reason. Their chronological age increases but their emotional age remains the same, and they continue to exhibit certain immature homosexual behavior patterns. According to Bryan (1967), such persons are really not homosexuals but immature persons exhibiting homosexual behavior. In discussing the treatment of such persons, Bryan stated

> It is useless to try to educate them to a more mature level, because if that had been possible they would have educated themselves long ago. The reason why they are not achieving their higher level is because of some subconscious block to their progress which stands in the way, and this block is usually in the form of a negative hypnotic suggestion which prevents them from gaining the maturity they seek. It is therefore absolutely essential to the cure of these individuals to age regress them back to the time in which the block occurred which impedes their growing up process. [p. 14]

This type of case is similar to the Ponce de Leon cases reported by Bryan (1964).

It is Dr. Bryan's contention that the most important etiological factor in homosexuality is the fear of death. It has been Dr. Bryan's experience that once the problem of survival has been solved, then the individual generally changes to heterosexuality easily and comfortably. The key to the problem is to find the cause of the disorder. Once the cause is uncovered, the rest will handle itself.

Some individuals exhibiting homosexual behavior need treatment and some do not. An individual who had several homosexual incidents at or near puberty doesn't need treatment for homosexuality in his adult years. Also, the individual isolated from heterosexual involvement over an extended period of time (military service, prison, etc.) needs no treatment other than aiding him in his proper placement in a heterosexual environment. There are, however, two categories of individuals exhibiting homosexual behavior who require treatment. These two categories are the immature individuals fixated at a specific developmental level emotionally while chronologically progressing, and individuals who accept homosexual behavior as the lesser of two evils when a life and death struggle is the alternative.

In discussing the handling of homosexuals, Bryan (1967) stated, "Persons exhibiting homosexual behavior should not be encouraged to adjust to it, but rather to be age regressed under hypnosis until the cause of their illness is uncovered and a cure has resulted." [p. 18] When we encourage a homosexual to adjust to his homosexuality, we are providing a means for adjustment to an emotional disorder rather than a cure for it.

Individuals falling into the category of fixation at an immature emotional level should be age regressed back to the time at which the subconscious block occurred, in the form of a negative hypnotic suggestion, which impeded their growing-up process. The negative hypnotic suggestion must be removed. The suggestion accepted by the patient always includes the false belief that it would be dangerous to grow up. Once the underlying fears and the subconscious hypnotic suggestions have been removed and replaced with positive suggestions (to the effect that from this moment he will be able to mature rapidly and completely in every way because there is no longer any reason to hold him back), then the patient is free to enjoy a normal aging process. He will generally rapidly adopt an adult heterosexual orientation.

Individuals who exhibit homosexual behavior because they have subconsciously accepted the suggestion that they couldn't survive as heterosexuals should be age regressed back to the particular time in their lives where the instinct for self-preservation was threatened and where the negative suggestion equating death and heterosexuality was accepted by the patient. Once the suggestion is removed by determining the underlying cause for its acceptance, heterosexual behavior will be adopted in most cases.

Chapter 24.

The Rip Van Winkle Syndrome: Hypnotherapeutic Treatment of Chronic Schizophrenics

The current trend within the field of mental health is to treat the mentally ill person in the setting in which his difficulties arose as well as to return hospitalized psychiatric patients to the community as soon as possible. The trend is also to reduce the population of the state mental hospitals, to discharge as many patients as possible. This is good, provided these people are adequately prepared.

Unfortunately, there are many chronic schizophrenic patients who have been hospitalized for lengthy periods of time and who are victims of the Rip Van Winkle syndrome because of the lengthy institutionalization. While the patient is in the hospital, the outside world changes, and in many cases he loses touch with his family and friends and forgets his old occupational skills and work habits. Treatment cannot be considered adequate or complete without recognition and resolution of the Rip Van Winkle syndrome, which is so prevalent within institutionalized mentally ill patients. I recognized this syndrome and was treating it without having a name for it. Then I recently read *Treating the Treatment Failures,* by Dr. Arnold Ludwig (1971), in which he used the term Rip Van Winkle syndrome in his discussion of the chronic schizophrenic.

There are three major phases to any comprehensive treatment program for chronic schizophrenics: (1) the modification of patient behavior within the hospital setting; (2) the preparation of patients for discharge; and (3) the provision for maintaining and rehabilitating discharged patients in the community. All three phases are mutually complementary, of relatively equal clinical importance, and of comparable difficulty.

This chapter will be devoted to the problems associated with the second of these phases. These problems pertain to many issues that have arisen about the best way of preparing patients to emerge from their institutional cocoons and to venture forth into the outside world.

Aside from dealing with the residual psychopathology present in predischarge chronic schizophrenic patients, the therapist must come to grips with many difficulties resulting from their prolonged hospitalization. Most of these difficulties are related to the Rip Van Winkle syndrome. In discussing the Rip Van Winkle syndrome, Ludwig (1971) stated:

> The patient, awakening from his long emotional and intellectual slumber, finds that the world outside the hospital is vastly different than when he was first hospitalized. During the years, there have been vast technological changes, well-known landmarks have disappeared, new buildings have been erected, transportation facilities have changed, and a myriad of other things have happened. The net result of his societal change and flux is that the outside world, in contrast to the relatively stable hospital environment, becomes a confusing, scary, and frightening place to explore for many patients. To borrow an analogy from the science fiction writers, it is as though patients were teleported by a time machine into an advanced, foreign civilization without possessing the necessary social skills or language for survival. [p. 192]

This situation is further complicated by the fact that during the course of prolonged hospitalization, many patients experience a deterioration in work habits, a diminution in self-confidence and self-discipline, an atrophy in social skills, the avoidance of competitive situations, a passive rather than active orientation toward the fulfillment of needs, and long exposure to an environment that places minimal demands and pressure on them. To accentuate the feeling of social alienation even further, over the years friendships deteriorate, family members die and family ties weaken.

With all these factors operating, many chronic schizophrenic patients show little or no motivation for leaving the relatively secure hospital environment. The readmission rate of these patients is very high because of their failure to cope in society. The longer patients are institutionalized, the more alien the outside world becomes.

If the relevance of the foregoing observations is accepted, it becomes readily apparent that this second phase of treatment is enormously important. The relevance and effectiveness of a predischarge program often makes the difference between a successful and an unsuccessful discharge.

In any adequate predischarge program, provisions must be made for enhancing patients' social and work skills, increasing their self-confidence in their ability to cope with new and often frustrating situations, increasing their self-discipline, increasing their level of motivation and helping them to feel that they are a part of the community at large. These are all formidable goals. To accomplish them in any degree, many innovative procedures have to be employed.

The following innovative hypnotic techniques may be effectively employed in predischarge programs for chronic schizophrenic patients.

The predischarge phase of treatment may utilize age regression in order to reconstruct prehospitalization attitudes toward work as well as to recall forgotten work skills and skills in interpersonal relations.

An audio tape recording that includes a progressive relaxation induction procedure as well as suggestions for strengthening the ego and for increasing motivation and self-confidence can be effectively employed in a group setting. Such a tape should be approximately twenty minutes in length and should be part of the daily predischarge program.

There are a number of uses of videotape that should be an integral part of the predischarge program. One important use of videotape would be to present a tape or a series of tapes that illustrate the following: instructions on reading a map of the city, demonstration of the correct use of a washer and dryer as well as other modern appliances, instructions on the use of the telephone book and a demonstration of the correct procedure for placing various types of phone calls (i.e., local, long distance, emergency), instructions on reading bus schedules, instructions on the completion of job application forms, a video guide of the city to include the state employment office, public library, city/county buildings, hospitals and clinics, YMCA/YWCA, bus depots, airports, shopping centers and centers of education and vocational training, and a video demonstration of job interviews, ordering food in a restaurant, buying a suit of clothes in a department store as well as any other situations that the discharged patient is likely to encounter.

Hypnodrama, a synthesis of psychodrama and hypnosis, is an extremely effective technique as part of a predischarge program. In hypnodrama, the protagonist, or main actor, acts out various roles while in hypnosis. The auxiliary egos or supporting actors may also be in hypnosis during the action phase of the drama. Hypnodrama may be utilized as a form of behavior rehearsal whereby patients are trained in necessary interpersonal skills and are given the opportunity to develop coping mechanisms and the ability to adapt to various roles within the community.

Training in self-hypnosis should be an integral part of the predischarge phase of treatment. Self-hypnosis may be used to reinforce suggestions for ego strengthening, self-confidence, relaxation and motivation. Age progression may be utilized in conjunction with self-hypnosis, whereby the person projects himself into the future and sees himself as already possessing all of the skills and personality traits necessary for successful living in the community.

In conclusion, it makes good clinical sense to develop a predischarge program geared to help chronic schizophrenic patients to overcome their basic deficiencies through active, participatory learning and to orient them to the world outside the hospital. In order for such a program to be effective, there should be ample utilization of hypnotic techniques before in vivo experiences are attempted.

Chapter 25.

The Treatment of Psychophysiologic Disorders by Hypnotherapy

When an underlying emotional difficulty is expressed through body systems innervated by the autonomic nervous system, the resulting condition is called a *psychophysiologic disorder.*

In his discussion of psychophysiologic disorders, Kisker (1964) pointed out that the etiology of psychophysiologic disorders is based upon four major factors: (1) constitutional sensitivity of the autonomic nervous system, (2) learning in the form of conditioning, (3) the symbolic advantage of a particular organ system, and (4) the presence of a stress situation. Every case of psychophysiologic disorder is ultimately dependent upon a combination of these four factors.

The hypnotherapeutic treatment of psychophysiologic disorders is similar to the hypnotherapeutic treatment of the other emotional disorders, except that the psychophysiologic disorders often require the additional attention of the medical specialist in the particular area of the physical symptom.

The treatment of the following psychophysiologic disorders by hypnotherapy will be presented: psychophysiologic cardiovascular disorders, gastrointestinal disorders, respiratory disorders, skin disorders, and genitourinary disorders.

PSYCHOPHYSIOLOGIC CARDIOVASCULAR DISORDERS

The cardiovascular reactions are among the most frequent of the psychophysiologic disorders and include essential hypertension and the postcoronary syndrome.

Stress due to repressed rage is considered an important factor in essential hypertension. Hypnorelaxation, posthypnotic suggestions, and sensory-imagery conditioning in a state of self-induced hypnosis are most effective in reducing high blood pressure. Self-hypnosis should be reinforced periodically.

Kroger (1963) has had gratifying results in a selected number of patients with postcoronary syndrome. Kroger stated that

> strong reassurance and reeducation under hypnosis directed toward achieving better adjustment to their condition, together with development of glove anesthesia, relieved or reduced their fears and anxieties and thereby raised their pain threshold. Those whose symptoms were ameliorated were advised to live within their limitations . . . Dietary control as well as salt reduction can be maintained by posthypnotic suggestions in those who have obesity, diabetes or hypertension. [p. 163]

In conjunction with hypnoidal desensitization, the patient is taught self-hypnosis and is encouraged to use self-exploration while in self-hypnosis to assess the degree of need for the symptom.

Most colitis sufferers have unresolved anxieties. The bowel becomes the target organ for displacement of unexpressed anxieties. The most satisfactory treatment approach consists of hypnorelaxation, sensory imagery, training in self-hypnosis, posthypnotic suggestions involving reassurance, a dietary regimen and tranquilizing drugs.

Gastrointestinal Disorders

The more usual gastrointestinal reactions are anorexia nervosa, or loss of appetite and weight, peptic ulcer and colitis, or inflammation of the colon.

Untreated cases of anorexia nervosa have a high mortality rate. It occurs chiefly in females who are very neurotic. Hypnosis can be utilized to keep the patient relaxed in bed and posthypnotic suggestions associating food with pleasant memories can be given to increase the appetite. Hypnosis can also be used to help the patient to ventilate feelings of aggression, hostility and guilt.

Most peptic ulcer patients will respond favorably to a treatment approach of hypnoidal desensitization, hypno-suggestion for symptom removal, training in self-hypnosis, reeducation and posthypnotic suggestions, when this treatment approach is incorporated within a medical regimen. The patient is asked to identify and enumerate all emotional situations connected with his symptoms in the order of their importance. A hierarchy of anxiety-arousing situations is constructed, beginning with the least anxiety-arousing scene and working up to the most anxiety-arousing.

RESPIRATORY DISORDERS

Bronchial asthma, tuberculosis and emphysema are examples of respiratory disorders which may be entirely or in part a result of emotional disturbance.

Asthmatic patients characteristically suppress all intense emotions involving threats to their dependent relationships. Hypnosis has been shown to be a useful method in the treatment of asthma (Collison, 1968; Hanley, 1974; Maher-Loughnan, 1970; Moorefield, 1971; Rose, 1967; Van Pelt, 1962). In adults, the disorder is often complicated by secondary psychological effects, such as chronic depression, or a defeatist attitude. The asthmatic patient may also derive secondary gain, which perpetuates the disorder.

The basic approach to the hypnotic treatment of the asthmatic patient, as presented by Hanley (1974), is for the therapist to analyze the emotional precipitants. The hypnotized patient is encouraged to explore and relate exactly what was happening, who he was with and what he was feeling just prior to a recent asthmatic attack and just before his first attack. The patient is then given suggestions of confidence, especially confidence that he can learn to control his own breathing. Then the patient is asked to produce an asthmatic attack and to stop it. This is repeated until the behavior has been learned. The patient is then taught self-hypnosis and is instructed to practice it daily and to use it whenever he does have an asthmatic episode. Patients are then seen at increasing intervals for reinforcement sessions.

While modern chemotherapy has revolutionized the treatment of tuberculosis, there are still a number of failures, and success still depends in large part upon the patient's cooperation, which is proportional to his ability to relax. Tuberculosis is in part a respiratory disorder of maladaptation due to stress. A large number of tubercular patients do not take their medication or leave the hospital prematurely. For those patients who require surgery, preoperative hypnosis can be useful in raising the threshold to shock. In those patients who require complete bed rest for months, hypnosis can facilitate relaxation and feelings of well-being. Hypnotic suggestions can be given to stimulate the appetite, promote sleep and to change any unhealthy attitudes the patient may have.

Emphysema is a respiratory disorder which is getting a great deal of attention today. Although it is a physical problem, it carries with it strong emotional connotations. When the patient has a great deal of difficulty breathing, he is filled with fear that the next breath may be his last. Hypnotic relaxation and hypnosuggestion can allay these fears and go a long way toward making the patient's life more comfortable. Since cigarette smoking plays a definite part in producing emphysema, hypnosis can be used to help the patient to stop smoking. A program for smoking withdrawal will be discussed in the chapter entitled "Group Hypnosis in Treatment."

Skin Disorders

The psychosomatic etiology for many skin disorders is well established. The skin is richly endowed with emotional symbolism. For example, "thick skinned" means insensitive, "thin skinned" means sensitive, and "itching to do something" means that a person can hardly wait to get on with it; if he isn't allowed to, it may actually result in feelings of scratchiness all over the body. The psyche rarely appears in dermatoses as the sole cause, but mental conflicts can be converted into skin disorders just as they can be converted into hysterical conversion and phobic disorders.

Hypnosis can be extremely valuable in the treatment of many skin disorders, such as acne vulgaris, eczema, neurodermatitis, psoriasis, and all forms of warts.

Hartland (1966) considered the following routine to be equally applicable in the hypnotic treatment of all psychophysiologic skin disorders:

> As a result of this treatment . . . you are going to feel physically stronger and fitter, in every way. Your circulation will improve . . . particularly the circulation through the little blood-vessels that supply the skin. (Here the doctor specifies the precise areas most

affected by the rash.) Your heart will beat more strongly . . . so that more blood will flow through the little blood-vessels in the skin . . . carrying more nourishment to the skin.

Because of this . . . your skin will become much better nourished . . . it will become healthier . . . more normal in texture . . . and the rash will gradually diminish . . . until it fades away completely . . . leaving the underlying new skin perfectly healthy and normal in every way . . . and . . . as your circulation improves . . . and your nerves become stronger . . . and steadier . . . so . . . they will become much less sensitive . . . much less easily irritated . . . Consequently . . . the itching and irritation will gradually subside and disappear . . . it will become less and less, each day . . . and you will no longer have any desire to scratch . . . If at any time . . . unknowingly . . . you do begin to scratch . . . the moment your fingers touch your skin . . . you will immediately realize what you are doing . . . and you will be able to stop yourself . . . before you have done any damage at all to the skin . . . Because of this . . . you will not only feel much less irritation and discomfort . . . but your skin will heal . . . and your rash will disappear, much more rapidly. Even if you should start to scratch in your sleep, at night . . . the moment your fingers touch your skin . . . you will wake up immediately and realize exactly what you are doing . . . And . . . because of this treatment . . . you will be able to exercise enough control to stop yourself, immediately . . . before you have done any damage to your skin. [pp. 270, 271]

In addition to the routine suggestions for skin conditions presented by Hartland, individuals suffering from psoriasis benefit a great deal from the sensory-imagery conditioning for psoriasis described by Kline (1955). The patient is told that he will be able to feel warm sensations throughout his body. Then he is told that he will be able to experience cold sensations throughout the body. Having experienced these, he is told that he will be able to feel sensations of heaviness, lightness, constriction and expansion, in all the areas of his body where he has the psoriasis. Then he is told that he will be able to feel warm sensations only in the areas where the psoriasis is, but not in the other areas of his body. Following this, he is told that he will experience cold sensations, but only in the lesion areas. This is followed by suggestions of localized sensations of lightness, heaviness, constriction and expansion. Thus a regular treatment sequence of hypnotic sensation is developed: warmth, cold, lightness, heaviness, constriction and expansion, followed finally by normal sensation and relaxation. Posthypnotic suggestions may then be given for experiencing this pattern of sensations daily at a time when he would be going through the induction of self-hypnosis. In addition, the patient is told that several times a day, whenever it might be convenient, he will be able to visualize the areas of his body which have lesions and he will be able to visualize them as if they are going through the sequence of induced sensations.

In the hypnotic treatment of warts, it is desirable to induce as deep a hypnotic state as possible. While it is not absolutely essential, the deeper the hypnosis, the more rapid will be the results. The following routine suggestions for the treatment of warts have been presented by Hartland (1966):

> As I stroke your hand . . . you can feel a feeling of warmth, spreading into the skin of your hand . . . As I go on stroking . . . that feeling of warmth is increasing . . . so that you can now feel it quite clearly . . . As soon as you can feel this sensation of warmth . . . please lift up your other hand." (The doctor continues to stroke, and to suggest the sensation of warmth, until he sees the hand rise.) "Good! Now put it down again! . . . And now . . . I am beginning to stroke the warts, themselves . . . And . . . as I stroke each of these warts . . . you will feel that the warmth is becoming concentrated in the warts . . . and that the warts are feeling warmer than the rest of your hand . . . Very good! Put it down again! . . . As that warmth spreads into your warts . . . they will gradually become smaller . . . they will begin to shrink . . . they will become flatter . . . and will gradually disappear . . . With every treatment . . . your skin will become healthier . . . the roots of the warts will shrivel . . . and the warts themselves will gradually wither away. [pp. 274, 275]

GENITOURINARY DISORDERS

The effect of the emotions on the genitourinary system is a common observation. Many cases of enuresis, urinary retention, menstrual disorders, and disturbances of sexual function have an emotional basis.

Postoperative urinary retention can often be completely relieved by posthypnotic suggestions (Brown, 1959). Kroger (1963) gives the following suggestion: "Perhaps you may be able to remember in detail what it felt like the last time you urinated. Try and imagine the sensations you experienced the last time you emptied your bladder." [p. 240] When possible, the patient is asked to describe the subjective sensations associated with the act of urinating. These are fed back immediately and during subsequent sessions. No time limit for carrying out the act is given. The patient is then trained in self-hypnosis and is told: "If you imagine yourself urinating again and again, then you will have no trouble starting the stream. Try not to urinate until you have reexperienced urinating in your mind first." [p. 240] Confidence replaces irrational fears as the result of the rehearsal of urinating under self-hypnosis.

Hypnosis has been used successfully by a number of practitioners for the treatment of enuresis (Bryan, 1960; Gilbert, 1957; Koster, 1954; Kroger, 1963; Solovey and Milechinin, 1959). Before instituting a program of hypnotherapy, the presence of physical problems such as kidney infection, a small bladder capacity, and diseases of the nervous system must be eliminated.

In many cases, the symptom of enuresis is the manifestation of a passive-aggressive interplay between child and parents. Once the child realizes that he has a weapon that he can use against his parents, he may maintain a conditioned response long after the cause for his hostility is forgotten. When this conditioned reflex becomes firmly established, the harder he tries not to wet the bed, the more likely he will be to lose control during sleep. Even though it is used as a passive-aggressive act, the child is ashamed of bed-wetting. However, he is not motivated to give up the secondary gain that the enuresis affords. The mother often resorts to nagging, which in turn makes the child more frustrated. In dealing with this situation, the parents must be treated concurrently with the child.

Since the child who presents himself for treatment of enuresis is usually very nervous and has been brought for the initial session against his will, rapport must be established immediately. A thorough history should be taken from the parents and then the child can be seen individually for a complete history and physical examination. After hypnosis is achieved, the child is asked if he enjoys wetting the bed. If a negative response is forthcoming, he may be asked how many of his classmates wet their beds. This indirectly helps to establish motivation for change. Then the child is asked how he would feel if he had an accident while sleeping overnight at a friend's house who didn't wet his bed. If he admits that this would be embarrassing, he is then asked whether he would like to be helped to avoid this situation in the future.

These questions serve a dual purpose. They focus the child's attention on the fact that he has a problem without making him feel guilty. They also reveal his personality structure and the most appropriate therapeutic approach. If the child is aggressive, a permissive approach may be used. If the child is passive, he can be encouraged to assert himself and to vent his resentments on the therapist and later he can be taught how to channel his aggression into more constructive outlets.

Then the child's feelings regarding his parents are explored. The therapist proceeds with analysis to get at the underlying cause of the enuresis. Even when the underlying cause is discovered and worked through, in many cases the habit pattern established is so strong that the enuresis will remain, even though the original cause has been removed. When the enuresis continues after analysis, rehabilitation techniques should be utilized to break the habit pattern.

One such technique is to strengthen the muscles surrounding the urethral orifice, thereby preventing bed-wetting on a neuromuscular basis. This is accomplished in two ways: (1) by having the patient start and stop three or four times every time he urinates; and (2) by letting the muscles around the urethral orifice contract as all other muscles relax (this is done with the patient in hypnosis). Another effective technique is drying the bed in stages. The child is asked while in hypnosis whether he would be interested in how much of his bed can remain dry. It can be suggested to the child that he controls his own bladder and that he can have a dry bed if he wants it badly enough. Never speak of bed-wetting but only of bed drying. The child's mother is instructed always to speak in terms of a dry bed. By continuing with this positive approach, the patient may be asked when he will be able to keep his bed completely dry all the time. He will then set a goal for himself which he will be able to keep quite accurately. The use of a calendar to mark off the nights when the bed was dry helps to strengthen the sense of achievement.

The onset of menstruation is tinged with emotion. All races exhibit guilt over this phenomenon and attempt to explain it through taboos and rituals. This natural phenomenon continues to be thought of by many people as disgusting and dirty. Therefore, it is not difficult to see how an unhealthy concept of menstruation can be formed early in life. The young girl at puberty may experience the passing of blood, and if not informed, she is forced to form her own opinion, often a distorted and frightening one.

A description of the following menstrual disorders will be given along with the most appropriate form of hypnotherapeutic treatment: premenstrual tension, functional dysmenorrhea, functional amenorrhea, and menopausal anxiety.

Before the onset of each menstrual period, there is usually an emotional reaction in women which is referred to as premenstrual tension. Some women become very moody and may show anxiety symptoms of varying degrees of severity. The symptoms usually disappear at the beginning of menstruation, but in some cases the symptoms are aggravated during the menstrual period. Such symptoms may involve resentment in connection with the feminine role.

During the premenstrual state in women suffering from premenstrual tension, the tension builds up gradually, with increasing restlessness, inability to concentrate, unreasonable emotional outbursts, crying spells without provocation and increased irritability and annoyance over trifles. These emotional changes may be accompanied by headache, backache, and insomnia.

Some of the underlying causes for premenstrual tension include resentment of the feminine role, hidden marital problems, and the fear of pregnancy. While the condition occurs in women without neurotic symptoms, the disorder is more common and much more severe in women with a neurotic character structure. If the woman is suffering from a psychoneurotic disorder, then the neurosis should be treated directly in hypnoanalysis, as the premenstrual tension is merely symptomatic of the neurotic framework.

Ideomotor questioning should be used to determine whether there are any underlying causes indicative of an active psychological conflict. If so, the patient should be treated in hypnoanalysis. The underlying cause should be discovered and worked through at an emotional level.

Functional dysmenorrhea is a common complaint and means pain with menstruation of such a degree as to cause the individual to be incapacitated. The causative factors in functional dysmenorrhea are psychogenic rather than organic.

Most cases of functional dysmenorrhea yield readily to hypnotic suggestion because dysmenorrhea often arises solely as a conditioned response without any underlying emotional conflicts.

The first step in the treatment of dysmenorrhea is the elimination of any organic cause. When the main cause of dysmenorrhea is found in previous conditioning, it will yield to direct symptom removal. While in hypnosis, it is suggested to the patient that menstruation is normal, and that every normal, healthy woman has periods. An increase of blood flow into the pelvic region and around the womb just prior to and during a period causes a feeling of congestion. Many women suffering from dysmenorrhea interpret this feeling of congestion to mean pain. Because they expect pain, they become tense and, consequently, the menstrual flow must be forced out; this results in additional pain.

As a result of direct hypnotic suggestion, the patient whose dysmenorrhea is due to previous conditioning will no longer interpret the feeling of congestion to mean pain, will be able to relax, and will be secure in the knowledge that having periods indicates that she is healthy and mature. She will lose all fear of having periods and will be able to relax during menstruation.

If symptom removal by direct suggestion fails, the symptom is most likely the physical manifestation of a more deep-seated emotional conflict which can best be dealt with by hypnoanalytical methods aimed at uncovering a more fundamental basis for the complaint. After the factors subjectively believed important in making the first painful menstrual period have been uncovered, the patient is age regressed back to the first painful menstruation and relives the feelings she experienced at that time. Then she is asked to turn off the pain at a subconscious level and have an ideomotor signal indicate completion and report verbally when she feels comfortable. The patient is then asked if it will be all right for her now to menstruate scantily three days each month and with complete comfort to do any of the things she would like to do when she is not menstruating. Such helpful suggestions in the form of a question reveal resistance due to unresolved self-punitive attitudes. If painful menstruation occurs after acceptance of these suggestions, previously undiscovered emotional factors must be found and worked through.

Before the termination of therapy, the patient should be told that there will be times when dysmenorrhea may occur again during an illness or a time of depression or emotional stress. At these times she should think of this "slip back to an outgrown habit" as a reminder to ask herself about and learn the factors responsible. In recognizing the factors involved, she will be able to turn off the pain with the techniques learned in therapy.

The diagnosis of functional amenorrhea is made in the absence of organic, endocrine, or nutritional factors. It may vary from a total cessation of the menses to a decided scantiness of the blood flow. Some psychogenic factors to be considered are: anxiety, shock or accident, death of a loved one, fear of pregnancy, faulty attitudes toward sex, emotional tension provoked by argument, change of climate and/or occupation, deprivation of male society and the wish to get pregnant (pseudocyesis). Also, fear of an unwanted pregnancy may produce functional amenorrhea. A complete history of each case is extremely important. Basic causations must be elicited.

Direct suggestion in hypnosis will often effect a complete cure. Dunbar (1938) stated:

> In many cases amenorrhea can be cured by one hypnotic session. In a patient who had been suffering from amenorrhea for two-and-one-half years, menses were induced by hypnosis, and regulated to occur on the first day of each month at 7 A.M. to last for three days. [p. 335]

In obstinate cases, or those in which the conflict is deep seated, hypnoanalysis should be employed, thus enabling the patient to gain insight into the factors responsible for the symptom-complex. In discussing the use of hypnotic age regression in the treatment of amenorrhea, Kroger (1963) stated: "The patient is regressed to her last period and asked to recall the specific sensations associated with it; if she wishes, she can choose the approximate date for the establishment of the menses." [p. 207]

Just as the individual passes through a critical phase in development at puberty, many women also become emotionally upset and anxious at the menopause. The symptoms of menopausal anxiety are often multiple and include vague lower abdominal pain, feelings of fullness, vaginal pain or irritation, and flushing. Because the factors underlying the complaints may be so diverse and because the symptoms may be so varied, each patient must have an individual approach. However, in the broadest terms, "hypnotic suggestions are offered which are calculated to calm the patient, to reassure her, to bolster up her self-confidence, to encourage her to face up to her problems, and by direct suggestion to remove her symptoms." (Leckie, 1964 p. 136) When this approach is ineffective, some deeper motive is sought by hypnoanalytic techniques and, when uncovered, this is dealt with.

Psychic impotence, premature ejaculation, and frigidity are the three most common disorders of sexual function. Two other rather common disorders of sexual function are psychogenic sterility and dyspareunia. Since the underlying psychodynamics and treatment approach are essentially the same for psychic impotence and premature ejaculation, they will be discussed together.

Organic frigidity is rare but should be clinically ruled out before treatment by hypnotherapy is initiated. Furthermore, it should be determined whether it is actually a case of pseudofrigidity due either to male or female ineptness or ignorance of sexual matters. If so, it can be treated by proper reeducation of attitudes of the male or female, or both.

The psychological cause of the frigidity must be fully explored. If the frigidity is a defense of a latently homosexual woman against a relationship with which she is emotionally unable to cope, it is a clear contraindication for hypnotherapy. If hypnosis is attempted with such a patient, an acute anxiety reaction may result.

Results and methods of treatment of frigidity will vary according to a woman's classification in one of the four major groups as outlined by Cheek and LeCron (1968). Group 1 (F) has never had an orgasm when awake or asleep, doesn't know what an orgasm should feel like, and has never knowingly masturbated. Group 2 (F-1) has had orgasms in dreams, with masturbation or with petting, but never during intercourse. Group 3 (F-2) has had orgasm with intercourse at one time, but not any more. Group 4 (RF) refers to relative frigidity estimated on a percentage basis in relation to times of intercourse. Individuals included in this group are classified with a number, i.e., RF 20 (percent) at the beginning of therapy.

Group 1 patients have no basis on which to judge experience, and therefore are the most difficult to treat. Women in this group often come from broken homes or homes where there was little display of affection. Cheek and LeCron have speculated that they probably had little skin stimulation during infancy. Their psychosexual developmental stages have been blocked at every turn. These patients should be placed in deep hypnosis and age regressed back to the birth experience; the therapist should check for and correct any misunderstandings that may have occurred at that time. Then they should be led to hallucinate the necessary steps of learning that have had no chance to occur. Cheek and LeCron included the following experiences:

> Being fondled and hugged by mother and father, discovering that it feels good to have the genital area cleaned and dusted with powder, that it feels good and is all right to slide down bannisters, that it is normal to explore the pleasurable feelings of masturbation. A search must be made for traumatic experiences with male relatives, old and young, and guilt feelings removed. [p. 119]

Then Cheek and LeCron ask for visual hallucinations of Christmas tree lights in various parts of the body representing the sensory awareness in these parts. These can be recognized at an ideomotor level and then elevated to a speaking level and reported. The patient is then asked to let the thought come into her mind of what color her breasts should be to be sensitive to caressing and what color the genital area should be for her to be able to reach a climax eight or ten times with intercourse. The patient is then asked to hallucinate forward to the time when these changes will have occurred, after she has removed all the guilt feelings and fears that have interfered with the capabilities she was born with. Failure to select a date indicates resistance to therapy and must be discovered and worked through.

At the next session, the patient is asked for a review of dreams and events since the last time she was in the office, to see if there were any moments when sensations in her body were similar to the chosen ideals. She is then age regressed back to about 13 years of age and told to pick up the normal type of dream of being fondled and of noticing pleasurable sensations in her breasts and clitoral area. She is asked to have an ideomotor signal if and whenever she has a subconscious feeling that approximates what she believes an orgasm might feel like.

The course of therapy from this point depends on information presented. It should be made clear to the patient that there are conscious feelings she will have at an appropriate time with the real experience, but that now she is being asked only for subconscious feelings which act like blueprints for the total feelings when the situation calls for these.

Patients in the other three groups offer much less of a problem and are handled in the same general way. First, it is determined through ideomotor questioning whether there is subconscious willingness to be helped with the problem and whether there is any real or imagined cause for the difficulty as it is now presented. Then the patient is aided in

> subconscious rehearsals of helpful dreams and real experiences with successive increasing loss of fears and inhibitions until there is ideomotor indication that orgasm can be reached with kissing, caressing of the breasts, entrance of the penis into the vagina, continued alternate contracting relaxation of the vagina around the penis and at any time there is an awareness of pulsating enlargement of the penis with ejaculation. [Cheek and LeCron, 1968 p. 121]

Although relatively few women will be able to achieve these goals in reality, subconscious awareness of the possibilities teaches them that orgasm is a mental process that doesn't need any specific stimulation to a target area. The fact that the patient is able to experience orgasm with dreams and hallucinated experiences in hypnosis convinces her that orgasm is a mental process.

Kroger (1963) referred to premature ejaculation and impotence as the "emotional plague" because they are so widespread in our culture.

The possibility of organic impotency should be ruled out before attempting hypnotherapy. A careful and thorough history must be taken before deciding on the treatment approach. The psychological causes of impotency may be due to anxiety produced by faulty attitudes toward sex, fear of failure, fatigue or repeated episodes of failure, hostility, and lack of affection, prolonged abstinence, a too aggressive or experienced sex partner or a sex partner who shows revulsion for the sex act or who has the desire to "get it over with." Impotency due to the aforementioned causes is usually successfully treated by means of attitude therapy and direct hypnotic suggestion.

If the impotency is due to a deep-seated need to fail in order to reject the wife, then hypnoanalysis will be necessary.

If the impotence is a symptom of latent homosexuality, treatment by hypnosis is contraindicated and the patient should be treated by a form of waking psychotherapy.

There should be a search for key or imprinted experiences in childhood and inhibiting factors should be searched out and removed before rehearsal of experiences as they should be. The patient should be placed in one of the four categories as devised by Cheek and LeCron for frigidity and should be treated from the same viewpoint.

Patients who suffer from psychogenic sterility are often anxious to have children and frequently express their disappointment in being unable to conceive. Consequently, intercourse is usually an anxiety-provoking situation for these women. Giving advice about precoital douching, special positions for coitus, etc., is ill advised because it will tend to make intercourse an even more stressful situation. Hypnotic relaxation and direct hypnotic suggestion usually proves to be an ideal method in treating psychogenic sterility. If this is unsuccessful, hypnoanalysis is called for. The husband and wife should both be seen in order to determine whether there are any inner tensions or emotional problems in the marriage. Hypnoanalytic techniques are utilized in order to determine why the idea of pregnancy is being rejected, either by the husband or the wife, or both. When the cause of the pregnancy rejection is determined and exposed to the patient at the conscious level, the condition will then usually yield readily to suggestions given in hypnosis. Posthypnotic suggestions of relaxation during intercourse are given. Positive suggestions of pregnancy are also implanted in the patient's mind in order to counteract the negative ones which she has probably held.

Dyspareunia refers to difficult and painful coitus. In discussing the factors that may be at work in dyspareunia, Leckie (1964) included the following:

> . . . misinformation (often amounting to fantasies) about the sex act, fear of pain related to coitus (especially of rupture to the hymen), ignorance of the female reproductive anatomy, ignorance and fantasies regarding the mutual adaptability of the male and female sex organs, and lack of any imaginative approach to the physical techniques involved in coitus may frequently be found, singly or in combination, to be, at least superficially, behind the complaint. [p. 129]

The best approach to the treatment of dyspareunia is hypnoanalysis followed by reeducation and direct hypnotic suggestion. Hypnoanalytic techniques such as age regression, induced dreams, sensory hypnoplasty and hypnography are employed in order to determine the cause of the condition. Then when the cause is determined and exposed to the patient at the conscious level, it is usually still necessary to employ interpretation, reeducation and direct hypnotic suggestion.

In hypnosis it is suggested to the patient that sexual intercourse between husband and wife is a normal, clean act which gives happiness and satisfaction to both husband and wife. It is further suggested that she has lost all fear of intercourse and that she is able to relax and that she can give herself completely to her husband as he gives himself to her.

Chapter 26.

Hypnotherapeutic Approaches to the Treatment of Alcoholism

The purpose of therapy with the alcoholic is to motivate the individual to stop drinking and then teach him how to adapt to his problems rather than using regressive behavior patterns at the first sign of stress. A sympathetic, noncondemnatory attitude makes the alcoholic feel that he is being treated like an adult and this helps establish healthy motivation.

Since most alcoholics are generally dependent, the hypnotic relationship initially helps the patient in therapy at a time when he is most resistant. Later this dependency is dissolved and the needs for it are worked through. Because of greater rapport with the therapist, the patient is willing to trade his self-destructive tendencies and immature attitudes for healthier and more realistic goals.

The successful treatment of alcoholics through the use of hypnosis depends on a thorough and complete management of the case. First of all, a complete physical examination of the patient should be conducted in which all diseases secondary to alcoholism, such as malnutrition, cirrhosis, etc., are correctly treated with the proper medication. This may require a period of hospitalization in which the patient cannot procure alcohol. It is vitally important that during hospitalization the patient be watched carefully so that alcohol is not brought to him by friends, relatives, or employees.

When the alcoholic leaves the hospital, he usually swears that he will never take another drink. It is at this time that the alcoholic is frequently in a good state of mind to get well, but too often he is just giving lip service to the many promises and good intentions without really meaning to do very much about them. In other words, although the alcoholic may have a conscious desire to stop drinking, at this point he has only been "dried out"; he still has the personality structure that led to the alcoholism and the habit pattern of heavy drinking.

The chronic alcoholic who doesn't wish to be helped, or who is brought in by friends or relatives against his will, cannot be helped by any psychotherapeutic approach unless he is institutionalized for long-term therapy. The prognosis is usually poor as each recovery is only a "flight into health."

Van Pelt (1958) referred to the vicious cycle created by alcoholism and pointed up the importance of finding the root cause of the neurosis that is responsible for the alcoholism. It is this phase of the treatment that few physicians are willing or adequately trained to undertake.

According to Bryan (1961), another reason for the failure in the treatment of many alcoholics is a failure on the part of the doctor to realize that there are two factors, both of which must be eliminated in order to permanently cure the alcoholic. The first factor is the root cause of the neurosis, or the cause of the compulsion to drink (it is usually multiple). The second is the powerful habit pattern established by the alcoholic through years of drinking.

The remainder of this chapter will deal with the various treatment approaches that utilize hypnosis with alcoholics. The first approach to be discussed is Dr. William J. Bryan's system of hypnoanalysis. Successful treatment of the alcoholic, according to Bryan, depends on following what he called the basic five R's of hypnotic treatment.

The first R is relaxation: the subject must be relaxed so that adequate communication can take place between the therapist and patient. The second R is realization: the patient must be made to realize the cause of his drinking. The causes of alcoholism are, Bryan felt, always multiple. He felt that it is essential to age regress the alcoholic to the period of each damaging experience and enable him to relive those experiences with the subsequent catharsis necessary to rid him of the hypnotic suggestion under which he is operating. In the treatment of alcoholics it is Bryan's policy to age regress patients right back to the first time they took a drink, the first time drinking became a problem for them, and every subsequent binge thereafter, if possible. It is frequently discovered what types of episodes seem to trigger off the alcoholic's desire to retreat from society into the security of liquor. After all of the underlying causes have been discovered, the patient has a catharsis for each damaging experience, and the negative emotions and suggestions associated with each event are removed.

Then the next phase of treatment is entered, employing the third R: reeducation, in which the patient is shown the relationship between the underlying causes and his drinking behavior. This phase also involves a change of attitude toward stress and problem areas in the alcoholic's life. Even though the root causes may have been discovered, the catharsis may have been obtained, and the compulsion to drink may be gone; nevertheless, a forceful habit pattern may still remain. In other words, even though the patient has no compulsion to drink, he has still been conditioned to a habit pattern over a long period of time, and may therefore continue to drink (automatically turning in at the first sign labeled BAR). The fourth R in Bryan's system of hypnotherapy is rehabilitation. The true rehabilitation of the alcoholic consists of breaking the habit pattern and strengthening the ego. The habit pattern can be broken in two ways, either by eliminating it entirely, or by substituting another habit pattern for the consumption of alcohol.

Bryan stressed the fact that unless the compulsion to drink has been completely taken care of under the first three steps of hypnotherapy, the substitution of a new habit pattern will not be sufficient to deter the alcoholic from drinking. The fifth R of Bryan's system of hypnotic treatment is reinforcement; this phase consists of seeing the alcoholic at regular intervals after the completion of hypnotherapy proper for the reinforcement of suggestions previously given. By individualizing the treatment of the patient suffering from alcoholism through the use of hypnosis, both diagnostically and therapeutically, with the five R method of treatment, Bryan claimed to have a 90 percent cure rate.

Conditioned reflex treatment (Lemere, 1959) has been successful for some alcoholic patients. In this approach, the patient is given a drink and an emetic is then administered. An association between vomiting and drinking is produced, but it isn't helpful unless the patient is highly motivated or is seen immediately after a hangover. Relatively permanent results have been obtained in carefully selected patients by reinforcing this technique through posthypnotic suggestions to vomit at the sight, taste or smell of liquor (Kroger, 1942). Motivation is increased by such posthypnotic suggestions as the setting of a deadline for the daily or weekly decrease in the quantity consumed and the stressing of the health factor, as well as by the effect of the patient's self-esteem that has been enhanced by the permissiveness of the therapeutic regimen. The key points in the conditioned reflex hypnotic treatment approach outlined by Wolberg (1948) is based on repeatedly emphasizing, under hypnosis, the bad effects of alcohol, the conditioned repugnance for alcoholic beverages and the patient's ability to control his own behavior, and establishing the emotional needs for the symptom.

Wolberg described an interesting technique in which symptom substitution is utilized. He informs the patient that "every time you crave a drink you will reach for a malted milk tablet, and this will give you a sense of pleasure and relaxation."

Kroger (1963) found that the results in small groups are often better than with individual hypnotherapy in the treatment of alcoholics. In addition to hypnosis, Kroger made use of free discussion and expression of feelings, reeducation, reassurance, strong emotional support and thorough explanations of commonly encountered problems. Kroger felt that group hypnotherapy is often more effective in resolving the patient's guilt, anxiety, insecurity and fear than individual hypnotherapy, especially if the patient identifies with strong members of the group. The stronger the identification, the more the alcoholic will emulate those whom he admires.

Kroger's approach to group hypnotherapy consists of weekly two-hour sessions. Each session begins with a general discussion of alcoholism. Questions and answers pertaining to all aspects of drinking are conducted during the first half-hour. Then several former patients who have been helped by group hypnotherapy relate their experiences. One or more grateful "cured" patients describe how they were taught hypnosis; how, after observing improvement in other group members, they were more motivated to obtain similar results; how they were taught autohypnosis and how through hypnotic conditioning they finally developed a profound disgust for alcohol. Having a "cured" group member sincerely relate his feelings to the group, a considerable amount of hope rapidly develops, especially for the neophyte or the disbeliever. After the presentation of former patients, successfully hypnotized volunteers are given appropriate suggestions for producing disgust and a strong aversion for drinking. Since a specific disgust to taste and smell will vary from patient to patient, Kroger suggested that each patient be allowed to select his own. In successive sessions, the techniques of autohypnosis and sensory-imagery are inculcated into each person. Kroger found that the incidence of success was much higher when autohypnosis was employed. With this approach, the patient realizes that he must achieve the results through his own efforts. This is highly motivating and contributes to his self-esteem. The patient may use autohypnosis for purposes of relaxation, sensory-imagery, and reinforcement of posthypnotic suggestions.

In conclusion, Bryan's system of individual hypnotherapy, Kroger's system of group hypnotherapy, and the conditioned reflex and aversive conditioning approaches to the hypnotic treatment of alcoholics have been discussed. I feel that a combination of all of these approaches is the most effective treatment plan, beginning with detoxification and an aversive conditioning approach, followed by individual hypnotherapy, and terminating in group hypnotherapy that includes training in self-hypnosis.

Chapter 27.

The Use of Hypnosis in the Treatment of Drug Addiction

The personality structure of the "average" addict shows many of the same defects as those of the chronic alcoholic. The addict is usually oversensitive, dependent, lonely, lacking in self-esteem, and finds it difficult to tolerate frustration. In addition, self-pity is often a prominent feature of the addict's personality.

Hartland (1966) mentioned two distinct types of addiction: (1) that which occurs in people suffering from neurosis who try to control their tension and anxiety with drugs; and (2) that which occurs in people who resort to drugs for the "lift" and feelings of euphoria that they induce. In either case, once addiction has developed, a physical dependency upon the drug is established as a result of biochemical changes, which produce a craving for the drug. Kroger contended that an uncontrollable craving occurs in predisposed individuals even after a single exposure to a narcotic drug.

The most defensible classification in the light of available evidence is the classification by Ausubel (1964). He distinguished between three basic categories of drug addiction: primary addiction, in which opiates have specific adjustive value for particular personality defects; symptomatic addiction, in which the use of opiates has no particular adjustive value and is only an incidental symptom of behavior disorder; and reactive addiction, in which drug use is a transitory developmental phenomenon in essentially normal individuals influenced by distorted peer group norms. According to

Ausubel, the difference between primary and symptomatic addiction is mainly a difference in the specificity of the adjustive value of opiate-induced euphoria for the personality disturbance involved; whereas reactive addiction is adjustive for developmental and situational stress or for conformity needs in a peer group and not for a serious personality defect.

In Ausubel's classification, primary drug addiction includes all addicts with personality trends for which addiction has specific adjustive value. The following subgroups are delineated: (1) the inadequate personality and (2) anxiety and reactive depression states. Symptomatic drug addiction occurs primarily as a nospecific symptom in aggressive antisocial sociopaths. Drug addiction has no particular adjustive value for this type of person. It is only one symptomatic outlet for the expression of his antisocial and aggressive trends. Reactive drug addiction is essentially an adolescent phenomenon having no adjustive value for any basic personality defect. It is a response to transitory developmental pressures, a means of expressing aggressive antiadult feelings, and a means of obtaining acceptance in certain peer groups. Ausubel stresses the fact that not all adolescent drug addicts can be placed in the category of reactive addiction. Many (15 to 20 percent) are inadequate personalities, anxiety neurotics, or sociopathic deviates whose addiction begins in adolescence.

In making a diagnosis of drug addiction, using Ausubel's classificatory scheme, it must be remembered that the actual etiology is multiple in nature. In reconstructing the genesis of each individual case, such variables as availability and the attitudinal orientation of the culture as a whole, of the neighborhood and of the peer group must be carefully evaluated. A definitive diagnosis can only be made after obtaining a thorough psychiatric history and psychological examination.

Addiction to barbiturates and dexedrine is particularly susceptible to hypnotic treatment, according to Bryan (1967). Bryan stated that withdrawal symptoms can be curbed by direct suggestion and the judicious administration of medication. Hypnoanalysis is needed to eliminate the underlying neurosis, but the prognosis in these cases is good.

The results of therapy cases of addiction to the hardcore opiates (morphine, heroin(pantapon, etc.), on the whole have been poor. However, Bryan reported good results with these cases, provided that the following five conditions were present:

1. The patient himself must be well motivated in order for him to have any lasting benefits.

2. The patient must be under constant supervision.

3. The drug supply must be completely and permanently shut off from the patient.

4. An extensive hypnoanalysis must be done to uncover every significant neurosis, and direct suggestion must be given which will afford the patient new escape valves to replace the use of the opiates.

5. Most important, the patient must be seen a minimum of one or two hours daily until a complete cure is effected, and then hypnotic suggestion should continue until one is positively assured that recurrence is unlikely.

Hypnosis has been used to traumatize the drug addict against any use of a needle (Truman, 1971). In Truman's example, after the patient had gone through her withdrawal period, the posthypnotic suggestion was given that she was to be normal in all respects, but that if she or anyone else attempted to put a needle into her body at any place, she would have a violent physical reaction. She was also told that upon coming out of hypnosis she would not remember that this suggestion had been given to her. At the time of Truman's report, the patient had been successful for a period of six weeks. She had shot up with heroin on one occasion during that six-week period, but had gone into a violent stomach retching and vomiting when she put the needle into her arm. This was such a negative experience that she did not have any pleasant flash as a result of the heroin.

Kroger (1963) stated that autohypnosis is especially helpful for withstanding the disagreeable subjective sensations produced by withdrawal. In several refractory cases, he suggested that the addict use sensory-imagery conditioning to imagine that he is giving himself an injection or taking a drug orally while in hypnosis. When the patient can revivify the pleasurable effects of the drug, withdrawal is accomplished more readily.

Baumann (1970) used a technique with adolescent drug abusers consisting of the following steps: (1) history and physical examination with a sincere attempt at establishing rapport; (2) reliving of a previous "good trip" or happy drug experience; (3) having the patient develop the hallucinated drug experience into one which, in his or her own opinion, was more rewarding, more intense, and more profitable than the original. The advantages of such an approach are that self-induced hallucinated experiences are not against the law, they are free and totally under the subject's control, and thus provide the need for independence, without depriving the person of the kick, adventure or escape previously supplied by injection or ingestion of illegal, expensive drugs with unpredictable present or future effects.

A technique similar to the one developed by Baumann has been employed by Alvin Ackerman and myself (1971) as part of several 36-hour weekend encounter marathons with female drug addicts. Each group consisted of 32 subjects. The technique consisted of having the subjects lie down on mats with blankets and pillows. Then, with eyes closed, they were taken through a progressive relaxation induction that included deep breathing exercises. Then the subjects were told to visualize a scene that gave them the feeling of peace and contentment, to let the scene become as clear and vivid as possible, to enter into the scene, to become part of it and be completely surrounded by it. They were further told to experience everything about the scene—all of the pleasant sounds, the pleasant sights, the pleasant smells, the pleasant tastes, and pleasant touches —and to let the whole self be filled with the good feelings from being part of it. They were told that as they continued to be part of the scene, some suggestions would be given to them that would be very beneficial for them; that they were not to pay any particular attention to these suggestions, but to just let them float into their minds without any conscious effort. They were then given the ego-strengthening suggestions developed by Hartland (1966). After the ego-strengthening suggestions were given, they were told to go back to the last good "trip" they had and to relive it completely. They were told that every minute of clock time would seem like an hour while on their "trip." They were given ten minutes for their trip; the use of the time distortion technique made the ten minute trip seem like ten hours. At the end of the ten minutes, they were told that it was time for them to come back to the present time and place and that the operator was going to count from one to five and that with each number he counted they would feel much lighter, and more alert, and much more refreshed. At the count of five, they were told to open their eyes, sit up and feel the immense sense of mental clarity and physical well-being. The results thus far have been very encouraging.

Historically, drug abusers have been asked by society to give up what they "enjoy"—that is, a synthetic agent which permits temporary escape from the harsh realities of everyday life and the concomitant anxiety, which today arises from the middle class American dream based on hard work, delay of need fulfillment and competitive-aggressive relationships with others. It appears much more realistic to satisfy the needs of a drug abuser by substitution and addition of further pleasure rather than by deprivation of gratifications. Because the revivification of a good trip is legal and under the control of a professionally trained person, difficulties with the addict associating with criminal elements in order to procure drugs are largely eliminated.

Techniques for handling drug addicts by group hypnotherapy have been described by Ludwig, Lyle, and Miller (1964). Their study was conducted at the U.S. Public Health Service Hospital in Lexington, Kentucky with 22 male addicts. The authors believed that the hypnotherapeutic techniques that were most successful in eliciting positive responses were those that seemed more magical, more authoritative, and oriented more toward dealing with current, practical, reality problems. They found that insight oriented treatment held little meaning. Introspection was not one of these addicts' virtues; they viewed therapy as "getting something from the doctor." The authors felt that group hypnotherapy with addicts offers a number of advantages, especially for short-term treatment programs. It undermines most of the destructive griping which seems characteristic of many group meetings with addicts and allows group members to participate equally in all aspects of the treatment program. Group hypnotherapy also seems conducive for extending the duration of the therapeutic session beyond its ordinary limits by means of posthypnotic suggestions. The authors stated that group hypnosis has some severe limitations. It didn't prove useful as a method for dealing with deep insightful material.

Ludwig and Levine (1965) used a new treatment technique that employs LSD and hypnosis in the cure of drug addicts. The authors conducted a controlled study in which 70 drug addicts were randomly assigned to five brief treatment techniques employing LSD, psychotherapy, and hypnosis. The results of this study revealed that patients treated with the hypnodelic technique (LSD + hypnosis + psychotherapy) for a single session showed greater improvement than patients treated with a single session of (a) LSD + psychotherapy, (b) LSD alone, (c) psychotherapy, or (d) hypnotherapy, when evaluated two weeks and two months after treatment. The primary contribution of LSD, according to Levine and Ludwig (1966), is its ability to produce a mental state in which thoughts and feelings assume an exaggerated sense of meaning, importance, and significance. While under the influence of the drug, patients seem to have a prolonged form of "eureka" experience, whereby old ideas may be seen in a new light and new ideas are more readily accepted. These ideas, according to the authors, tend to become imbued with a new sense of intellectual and emotional appreciation. The addition of hypnosis to LSD increases therapeutic effectiveness for the following reasons:

1. Because of the hypnotic relaxation, the patient is better able to give in to the ensuing LSD experience.

2. During the hypnotic induction, the patient works closely with the therapist, and this relationship tends to be maintained throughout the LSD experience.

3. Because of the demand characteristics of the hypnotic situation, it is easier to structure, direct, and shape the session in ways the therapist deems important.

In conclusion, the use of hypnosis in the treatment of drug addiction shows a great deal of promise. Without the use of a long-range program utilizing hypnosis, the rate of success is around 2%. Success rates in programs employing hypnosis have consistently been between 60% and 70%. Group hypnotherapy, hypnodelic therapy and reliving a good trip, seem more likely to achieve results than hypnoanalysis, especially if they are employed in an institutional setting where treatment can be intensive, and where the addict can be kept under strict supervision. Other adjunctive therapies, such as drugs for withdrawal symptoms, vitamins, sedation, a nutritious diet, and occupational, industrial, and recreational therapy can also be helpful in conjunction with hypnotherapy.

Chapter 28.

Group Hypnosis in Treatment

Group hypnotherapy has been found to be an effective treatment method for such varied problems as obesity, smoking, anxiety, alcoholism and schizophrenia. The severity of maladjustment does not appear to be a precluding factor: group hypnotherapy has been utilized even with relatively regressed schizophrenics.

The composition of a hypnotherapy group may be of two types: according to symptomotology or varied composition. The use of group hypnotherapy lends itself to the typical group therapy session length of about an hour and one-half.

This chapter will deal with the use of hypnosis in the group therapy process as well as the use of hypnosis in specialized groups, such as weight control and smoking withdrawal.

Peberdy (1960) reported on hypnotic methods in group therapy. According to Peberdy, to have out-patient discussion groups is difficult, as many patients don't continue to show up or show up erratically; many don't like to discuss their problems, and group composition is always a problem. In this study, all patients had been suffering from morbid tension as a common theme and the major suggestions were of confidence and relaxation given with indications of posthypnotic continuance and reinforcement. The specific symptoms of some patients were alluded to in the suggestions when these would not be incongruent with the rest of the group. Groups composed of six patients each were given time before hypnosis to discuss their feelings, fears and impressions of group hypnotherapy. It was found that members often afforded each other invaluable support. The groups were composed of people in all stages of progress, and in general, individual hypnotic sessions were not required. Approximately 65 patients were treated. Detailed records of responses, reactions and results were kept. It was concluded that the patients' major symptoms of tension were much improved in 25% of the cases, reasonably improved in 25% of the cases and the rest were not aided.

That group hypnotherapy may be an effective method of treatment for psychoses is indicated by a study made by Ilovsky (1962). While the first group of schizophrenics treated consisted of 10 patients, he later treated groups as large as 150. This study reported on 80 chronic schizophrenic women whose average hospital stay was six to eight years. They were hypnotized twice weekly for six months both by the therapist and by a tape recording of the therapist's voice. Direct therapeutic suggestions were given to the patients by the therapist.

The author pointed out that hypnosis was especially useful with paranoid schizophrenics whose hostility could be controlled and directed through hypnosis to both socially and individually satisfactory channels. Ilovsky noted that the patients could be considered conditioned by suggestions to use their energy for working and repression instead of spending their time on expending aggression and hostility.

The results of this study revealed that at the end of the year, 60% of the patients treated were released from the hospital and that those remaining were considered more manageable. It was noted that the results with tape recordings were the same as those with direct personal hypnosis and that the rate of improvement was in direct proportion to the depth of trance achieved.

It has been found particularly effective to use a progressive relaxation induction technique in group hypnotherapy, beginning the induction with the eyes closed. This eliminates the possibility of a new client being primarily involved with observing the other clients, as well as providing an element of privacy for each client.

In her excellent paper on the use of hypnosis in the group process, Serlin (1970) reported that the kinds of material that may be readily elicited through the use of hypnosis in the group process include such areas as historical information about the patient, attitudes toward significant others, genuine feelings of love, rage, depression and anxiety, neurotic feelings and self-image.

Common to both individual and group hypnotherapy is the client's anxiety about the use of hypnosis. In both individual and group hypnotherapy, he fears loss of control; he has anxiety that something might be done to him that he is unaware of while he is in hypnosis; and he fears that he may reveal things to the therapist that he is not yet ready to reveal. In group hypnotherapy, the client has the additional concern that other group members will become aware of material about which he still feels a sense of privacy or fear of self-revelation. It is therefore extremely important that group participants are helped to achieve a complete sense of reassurance that whatever is experienced in hypnosis may remain a completely private experience. In order to alleviate this anxiety, it is helpful to emphasize prior to induction that the procedure does not involve any of the group members saying or doing anything while in hypnosis. It requires only that they think about certain things that the hypnotherapist suggests. Also, it should be emphasized that it will be entirely up to each individual at the termination of the hypnotic period whether or not he chooses to discuss any of the material he thought of while in hypnosis.

The most frequently used techniques for obtaining significant material in group hypnotherapy are generally identical to those techniques common to individual hypnotherapy. It may be suggested to the group members while in hypnosis that they have a dream about a particular area, that they recall particular incidents that relate to areas being investigated in the group process, or that they have thoughts that are associated with specific feelings. Revivification of past incidents may also be utilized. The subject suggested by the hypnotherapist may be that which has been under discussion during the group session prior to the induction of hypnosis, or it may be an area that is being avoided by the group.

Hypnosis may be introduced into the group process when it is felt that the material being examined is too peripheral or too superficial, or when there is group resistance. Upon termination of hypnosis, the therapist may ask who wishes to speak first. There is often spontaneous production of hypnotic material by the group members.

Insight into the defense mechanisms used by clients as well as into their genuine needs occurs primarily during the group discussion period. Hence, hypnosis is utilized primarily for the elicitation of material that can subsequently be subjected to scrutiny by the group.

It is highly desirable that the client leave the group therapy session with a feeling of the probability of success from therapy and hopefulness relative to his own success in achieving some of his goals in therapy. This may be accomplished by means of ego-integrative or supportive scenes in hypnosis with instructions to the client to visualize the happiest time of his life, or a time of complete joy or a scene of total success in handling a situation. The greatest value is from those scenes that have actually occurred in the client's own life.

In addition to the use of hypnosis in the group process, group hypnotherapy may be utilized in specialized areas, such as weight control, smoking withdrawal, concentration and examination behavior and hypnodramatic assertive training. I conducted specialized hypnotherapy groups in these areas over a two-year period in a university counseling center. A brief description of each group follows.

Before being accepted for the weight control group, each prospective group member was required to take the A-D Scale (a combination of the Taylor Manifest Anxiety Scale and the Depression Scale of the Minnesota Multiphasic Personality Inventory). If the person scored high on anxiety and/or depression, he was not accepted into the weight control group; instead, individual psychotherapy was recommended. Also, individuals were required to have a physical examination and permission from their physician prior to being accepted for the group. The weight control group included eight weekly one-hour sessions. During the first session, the misconceptions of hypnosis were discussed, and each client completed a form relating to eating habits and historical data pertinent to his overweight problem. A lecture period followed, and the session was concluded with a group hypnotic induction using the progressive relaxation technique. All lecture material for the weight control group was taken from Lindner's *Mind Over Platter* (1965).

A diet diary form was handed out at the second session, and the group members were told to list everything they ate each day, the time of day, and the approximate number of calories. They were told to follow their physician's instructions concerning calorie intake. The remainder of the second session was devoted to group induction of hypnosis, lecture (all lectures were conducted with group members in hypnosis), and a discussion with each group member about his eating habits and overweight problem with appropriate suggestions for correcting poor eating habits.

The third session included collecting the diet diary reports and giving a report of the number of pounds lost by the group during the previous week, group induction, lecture and ideomotor questioning, with each group member attempting to determine subconscious motivation and underlying causes of the overweight problem. An ideomotor questionnaire for overweight cases, consisting of 35 questions, was constructed by the author for use in the weight control group. The third session was concluded with group training in self-hypnosis, lecture, and a description of *Dr. Lindner's "Point System" Weight Control Program* (Lindner and Lindner, 1966). Each group member was given a copy of the book and told to begin using the point system rather than calorie counting.

The fourth session included diet diary reports, group induction, lecture, continuation of ideomotor questioning and group training in self-hypnosis. The fifth through the eighth sessions consisted of diet diary reports, reports on group weight loss, and the discussion of each group member's problems connected with overweight and overeating. Free ventilation was encouraged during this part of the session before hypnosis was induced. Then group hypnosis was induced and appropriate suggestions were given. The sessions ended with the group members going into self-hypnosis and arousing themselves.

The smoking withdrawal group was held for five weekly sessions; the sixth and seventh sessions were held bi-weekly. Prospective group members were required to have permission from their physician prior to acceptance into the group. The first session consisted of lecture material from *How To Stop Smoking Through Self-Hypnosis* (LeCron, 1964), a summary of the Surgeon General's Report, a discussion of the misconceptions about hypnosis and instructions for keeping a notebook that contained the following information: each time they smoked, the time of day, and what type of activity they were engaged in at the time. They were also given an assignment to write an autobiography of their smoking habit entitled "Why I Smoke."

The second session consisted of completing a questionnaire designed to determine whether the client is a light, medium or heavy smoker. This was followed by group hypnotic induction, instructions to the group members (instructions followed the 21-day program as outlined by von Dedenroth, 1964 a and b), ideomotor questioning to determine subconscious motivation and underlying causes of smoking and conditioning for self-hypnosis.

The third session consisted of group induction, lecture, suggestions to help stop smoking, further instructions (as per von Dedenroth's program), a discussion of notebooks and autobiographies with each client, and conditioning for self-hypnosis. The fourth session consisted of self-hypnotic induction, a lecture entitled "Your Program For Q Day" (quit day), suggestions to help stop smoking, and a discussion of notebooks with each client.

The fifth session began with immediate induction of the hypnotic state; the fact that good habits had already replaced bad habits was stressed and restressed. This was followed by a lecture entitled "Your Program After Q Day" and suggestions to help stop smoking. The sixth and seventh sessions were meant to be reinforcement sessions. A report on each group member's progress was made. Each group member's problems, if any, were openly discussed. Free ventilation was encouraged during that part of the session. Then hypnosis was induced and appropriate suggestions were given. The session ended with each group member going into self-hypnosis and arousing himself.

The concentration and examination behavior group consisted of four sessions. The first session included a discussion of the misconceptions about hypnosis, a progressive relaxation hypnotic induction, an ego-strengthening routine (Hartland, 1965), suggestions for improving concentration and study habits and for overcoming examination panic, and conditioning for self-hypnosis. The second, third, and fourth sessions consisted of progressive relaxation induction, ego-strengthening routine, and the first, second, and third scripts for deep concentration (Lieberman et al., 1968), one script for each session.

The hypnodramatic assertive training group was an ongoing weekly group and entrance was either by referral from another staff member in the counseling center or by self-referral. In deciding whether or not assertive training was indicated, prospective group members were given the *Assertive Interaction Questionnaire* (Wolpe and Lazarus, 1966), the *Willoughby Schedule* (Wolpe, 1958), and the *Historical Data Questionnaire* (Hartman, 1971). The person to whom assertive training applies has unadaptive anxiety-response habits in interpersonal relationships, and the evocation of anxiety inhibits the expression of appropriate feelings and the performance of adaptive acts.

The assertive training procedure usually commenced with a description of ineffectual forms of behavior in general and their emotional repercussions. Salter's *Conditioned Reflex Therapy* (1961) was assigned for its pertinent case history material. While being trained in assertive behavior, clients were told to keep careful notes of all their significant interpersonal encounters and to discuss them in detail with the therapist. It was necessary to know the circumstances of the encounter, the client's feelings at the time, the manner in which he reacted, how he felt immediately after the encounter, and his own subsequent appraisal of the situation. Upon the identification of debilitating inhibitions, the therapist firmly stressed assertive as opposed to aggressive reactions where applicable. A form of role playing known as behavior rehearsal is used by behavior therapists in assertive training.

I replaced behavior rehearsal with hypnodrama, which is a synthesis of psychodrama and hypnosis developed by J. L. Moreno. Dr. Moreno made a number of hypnodramatic experiments with Dr. James Enneis, the results of which they published in a monograph (Moreno and Enneis, 1950).

In hypnodrama, the personality structure of the protagonist can be split or dissociated for separate study—the protagonist can act out both roles. In this way the subject actually reenacts his own inner conflicts. Age regression and many other hypnoanalytic techniques can be used in conjunction with hypnodrama.

Assertive training is a teaching situation in which the client is taught to respond in an appropriate manner in those situations that call for some type of assertive response, whether it be voicing justifiable criticism or expressing affectionate feelings. The closer the teaching situation comes to approximating the real life situation, the greater the transfer should be from the practice session of being assertive to assertive behavior in vivo. This certainly was the case with those individuals I observed in hypnodramatic assertive training. This approach elicited a wealth of subconscious material which would not have been elicited with behavior rehearsal.

Part Seven
Research and Training
in Hypnotherapy

Chapter 29.

Individual Differences in Hypnotizability: Hypnotic Susceptibility Scales

The hypnotic susceptibility scale has specificity with respect to induction techniques and quantification of response that is lacking in the clinical depth scales, thus making this type of scale suitable for research purposes. The hypnotic susceptibility scales to be discussed are: the Stanford Hypnotic Susceptibility Scales, the Stanford Profile Scales, the Harvard Group Scale of Hypnotic Susceptibility, the Children's Hypnotic Susceptibility Scale, and the Barber Suggestibility Scale.

The clinical depth scales are suitable for strictly clinical purposes; however, if the hypnotic operator desires to perform comparative studies of hypnotic susceptibility, he should be familiar with the hypnotic susceptibility scales and use the one most suitable for his research purposes.

Dissatisfaction with the existing scales (i.e., clinical depth scales), led Weitzenhoffer and Hilgard to the development of the Stanford Hypnotic Susceptibility Scale. It was originally prepared in two forms. Form A and Form B were essentially equivalent forms to permit before-and-after studies (Weitzenhoffer and Hilgard, 1959). An additional form, Form C, was later added to meet new specifications (Weitzenhoffer and Hilgard, 1962). The Stanford Profile Scales were prepared to emphasize the differential aspects of hypnotic behavior (Weitzenhoffer and Hilgard, 1963; Hilgard, Lauer, and Morgan, 1963). Form A of the Stanford Hypnotic Susceptibility Scale was adapted at Harvard for group administration; this is known as The Harvard Group Scale of Hypnotic Susceptibility (Shor and Orne, 1962). London (1962) developed a scale closely related to the Stanford Scale for use with children; this is known as the Children's Hypnotic Susceptibility Scale. Barber developed a scale known as the Barber Suggestibility Scale (Barber and Glass, 1962). It is an eight-item scale to be used with or without prior hypnotic induction as a test of hypnoticlike behavior. All of these scales will be discussed separately.

STANFORD HYPNOTIC SUSCEPTIBILITY SCALES

These three scales were developed at Stanford University by Ernest Hilgard and Andre Weitzenhoffer. Forms A and B are essentially an expansion and refinement of the Friedlander-Sarbin scales, with similar inductions, many of the same items and a simplified scoring basis. The two forms, essentially equivalent, permit before-and-after studies. The items in Forms A and B are: postural sway, eye closure, hand lowering, arm immobilization, finger lock, arm rigidity, moving hands together, verbal inhibition, hallucination, eye catalepsy, posthypnotic suggestion, and amnesia. The content of Form C is somewhat richer than that of A or B, with more cognitive-type material (hallucinations, dreams, age regression).

STANFORD PROFILE SCALES, FORMS I AND II

In working with the earlier hypnotic susceptibility scales, it became evident that some highscoring subjects had clear gaps in their scores. For example, some who had high scores on the motor items failed to respond to posthypnotic amnesia instructions, whereas for others, the converse was true (Hilgard and Hilgard, 1962). According to Hilgard (1967), "It became clear that some sort of scale diagnostic of the special abilities associated with hypnotic performance would be valuable, a scale which minimized the common factor in hypnosis in favor of a profile of special abilities." The Stanford Profile Scales were standardized to meet this need. These scales yield a profile of scores instead of a single score of hypnotic susceptibility, thus showing areas of strength and weakness.

HARVARD GROUP SCALE
OF HYPNOTIC SUSCEPTIBILITY

This scale was developed by Ronald Shor and Emily Orne. It is a group adaptation of the Stanford Scale, Form A, arranged for self-scoring. The items are very similar to those of Form A of the Stanford Scales.

CHILDREN'S HYPNOTIC SUSCEPTIBILITY SCALE

This scale was developed by Perry London. It is designed especially for children, classified into two age categories (ages 5 years, 0 months through 12 years, 11 months; and ages 13 years, 0 months through 16 years, 11 months).

BARBER SUGGESTIBILITY SCALE

Developed by T. X. Barber, this scale differs from the Stanford Scales, the Harvard Group Scale and the Children's Hypnotic Susceptibility Scale in that it is intended to test hypnoticlike behaviors without prior induction of hypnosis. Objective and subjective scores are obtained for the following items: arm lowering, arm levitation, hands locked in lap, suggestion of extreme thirst, verbal inhibition, body immobility, posthypnotic response and selective amnesia.

The items and scoring criteria for each scale are presented in Tables 6 through 11.

TABLE 6.

STANFORD HYPNOTIC SUSCEPTIBILITY SCALE

Forms A and B (Weitzenhoffer and Hilgard, 1959)

Item	Form A	Form B	Criterion of Passing
1. Postural sway	Backwards	Backwards	Falls without forcing
2. Eye closure	Form A induction	Form B induction	Eyes close without forcing
3. Hand lowering	Left	Right	Lowers at least 6 inches bv end of 10 seconds
4. Arm immobilization	Right arm	Left arm	Arm rises less than 1 inch in 10 seconds
5. Finger lock	Before chest	Overhead	Incomplete separation of fingers at end of 10 seconds
6. Arm rigidity	Left arm	Right arm	Less than 2 inches of arm bending in 10 seconds
7. Moving hands	Together	Apart	(A) Hands close at least 6 inches
8. Verbal inhibition	Name	Home town	Name unspoken in 10 seconds
9. Hallucination	Fly	Mosquito	Any movement, grimacing, acknowledgement of effect
10. Eye catalepsy	Both eyes closed	Both eyes closed	Eyes remain closed at end of 10 seconds
11. Posthypnotic suggestion	Changes chairs	Rises, stretches	Any partial movement response at signal
12. Amnesia	Recall of items 3-11	Recall of items 3-11	Recall of three or fewer items

Total possible score: 12 points

TABLE 7.
STANFORD HYPNOTIC SUSCEPTIBILITY SCALE
Form C (Weitzenhoffer and Hilgard, 1962)

Item	Criterion of Passing
0. Eye closure during induction	(As in Form B, but not counted)
1. Hand lowering (right hand)	Lowers at least 6 inches in 10 seconds
2. Moving hands apart	Hands 6 inches or more apart after 10 seconds
3. Mosquito hallucination	Any acknowledgment of effect
4. Taste hallucination (sweet, sour)	Both tastes experienced and one strong or with overt movements
5. Arm rigidity (right arm)	Less than 2 inches of arm bending in 10 seconds
6. Dream	Dreams well; experience comparable to a dream
7. Age regression (school fifth and second grades)	Clear change in handwriting between present and at regressed age
8. Anosmia to ammonia	Odor of ammonia denied and overt signs absent
9. Arm immobilization (left arm)	Arm rises less than 1 inch in 10 seconds
10. Hallucinated voice	Subject answers voice realistically at least once
11. Negative visual hallucination (two or three boxes)	Reports seeing only two boxes
12. Posthypnotic amnesia	Subject recalls three or fewer items before being told, "Now you can remember everything"

Total possible score: 12 points

TABLE 8.

STANFORD PROFILE SCALES OF HYPNOTIC SUSCEPTIBILITY (SPS)

Forms I and II (Weitzenhoffer and Hilgard, 1963)

Form I: Induction by Hand Levitation (not scored)		Form II: Induction by Hand Lowering (not scored)	
1. Hand analgesia	0-3	1. Heat hallucination	0-3
2. Music hallucination	0-3	2. Selective deafness	0-3
3. Anosmia to ammonia	0-3	3. Hallucinated ammonia	0-3
4. Recall of meal	0-3	4. Regression to birthday	0-3
5. Hallucinated light	0-3	5. Missing watch hand	0-3
6. Dream I: topic unspecified	0-3	6. Dream II: about hypnosis	0-3
7. Agnosia I: house	0-3	7. Agnosia II: scissors	0-3
8. Joke	0-3	8. Personality alteration	0-3
9. Posthypnotic verbal compulsion	0-3	9. Posthypnotic automatic writing	0-3
Total	0-27	Total	0-27

TABLE 9.

HARVARD GROUP SCALE OF HYPNOTIC SUSCEPTIBILITY
(Shor and Orne, 1962)

Item	Criterion of passing
1. Head falling	Head falls forward at least 2 inches
2. Eye closure	Eyelids close before subject is told to close them deliberately
3. Hand lowering	Lowered at least 6 inches before told to let hand down deliberately
4. Arm immobilization	Hand not lifted more than 1 inch when told to stop trying
5. Finger lock	Fingers incompletely separated when told to stop trying
6. Arm rigidity	Arm bent less than 2 inches before being told to stop trying
7. Moving hands together	Hands not more than 6 inches apart when told to return them to resting position
8. Communication inhibition (headshake, "No")	Did not shake head before told to stop trying
9. Fly hallucination	Outward acknowledgment of effect
10. Eye catalepsy	Eyes remained closed
11. Posthypnotic suggestion (touches ankle)	Makes at least observable partial movement to touch ankle
12. Amnesia	Three or fewer items listed in 3 minutes, before amnesia lifted

Total possible score: 12 points

TABLE 10.

CHILDREN'S HYPNOTIC SUSCEPTIBILITY SCALE
(London, 1962)

PART ONE

Item	Minimum for plus score
1. Postural sway	Loses balance and recovers without falling
2. Eye closure	Eyes close within 10 seconds of final instruction before request to close eyes
3. Hand lowering	Hand moves through arc of 30 degrees or more
4. Arm immobilization	Hand rises from 1 to 3 inches, or with effortful movement, up to 4 inches
5. Finger lock	Incomplete separation of fingers, little effort
6. Arm rigidity	Arm bends less than 2 inches, with little effort
7. Hands together	Hands move to within 2 inches of each other
8. Verbal inhibition	Name not spoken; little effort
9. Auditory hallucination	Appropriate movement
10. Eye catalepsy	Eyes remain closed; little effort
11. Posthypnotic suggestion	Remains seated and stretches, or stands but does not stretch
12. Amnesia	Three or fewer items recalled with relative ease

TABLE 10.

Children's Hypnotic Susceptibility Scale (continued)

PART TWO

Item	Minimum for plus score
13. Posthypnotic suggestion (reinduction)	Closes eyes; eyes open but glazed
14. Visual & auditory hallucination	Sees TV set, turns it on; may fail to see picture clearly
15. Cold hallucination	Appropriate verbal response
16. Anesthesia	May be aware of stimulus, but unable to describe it
17. Taste hallucination	Experiences at least slight or vague taste sensations
18. Smell hallucination (perfume)	Affirms odor of perfume
19. Visual hallucination	Sees rabbit, describes it; may not pick it up
20. Age regression	Changes writing of name or figure drawing appropriately
21. Dream	Perfunctory report, but doesn't appear to be composing story during report
22. Awakening & posthypnotic suggestion	Sees rabbit posthypnotically

TABLE 11.
BARBER SUGGESTIBILITY SCALE (BSS)
(Barber and Glass, 1962)

Item	Scoring Criteria
0. Chevreul pendulum	Not scored
1. Arm lowering (eyes open)	1 point for 4 inches or more
2. Arm levitation from horizontally extended position (eyes open)	1 point for response of 4 inches or more
3. Hands locked in lap (eyes open)	½ point for incomplete separation after 5 seconds of effort or 1 point for incomplete separation after 15 seconds of effort
4. Suggestion of extreme thirst (eyes closed)	½ point for swallowing, lip moistening, etc. and ½ point for indication, during posthypnotic interview, that subject became thirsty
5. Verbal inhibition (name) (eyes closed)	½ point if name not said after 5 seconds of effort or 1 point if name not said after 15 seconds of effort
6. Body immobility (inability to stand up) (eyes closed)	½ point if not completely standing after 5 seconds of effort, or 1 point if not completely standing after 15 seconds of effort
7. Posthypnotic response (cough to a click) (suggested with eyes closed; tested with eyes open)	1 point if subject coughs to click
8. Selective amnesia (to remember all tests except arm moving up) (suggested with eyes closed; tested with eyes open)	1 point if subject recalls all other tests but Test 2 and recalls it in response to cue words

Total possible score: 8 points

Chapter 30.

Applied Research in Hypnotherapy

The system of hypnotherapy described in this book is an outgrowth of personal experience with many types of clients; it represents an integration and synthesis of the various approaches to hypnotherapy existent in the literature. Although a great deal of applied clinical research has preceded the development of my system of hypnotherapy in its present form, I view it as something dynamic, flexible and in need of constant revision in light of findings from ongoing applied clinical research.

The following data are gathered on every client seen for hypnotherapy:

STATISTICAL DATA

Age
Sex
Marital status
Educational level
Income level
Religious affiliation

HISTORICAL DATA

History and development of chief complaint:
    Chief complaint
    Date of onset
    Gradual or sudden onset

Severity of disorder

Number of previous consultations concerning chief complaint

Number of sessions of previous consultations

Family history:

    Father—occupation; if deceased, cause of death; general personality; attitude towards client

    Mother—occupation; if deceased, cause of death; attitude towards client

    Siblings—number, ages, marital status, and relationship of client with each

    Home atmosphere

    Ability to confide in parents

    Religious training

    Dominant family values and concerns

    Parent to whom client felt closest

    Method of parental punishment

Military history:

    Branch of service

    Highest rank

    Where stationed

    Dates of induction and discharge

Marital history:

    Length of present marriage

    Previous marriages—number and length

    Relationship with spouse

    Children—number and ages

Sexual history:

    Age at first sexual experience

    Parents' attitudes towards sex

    Disorders of sexual function—type and degree

Occupational history:

    Present occupation

    Length of time in present occupation

    Level of satisfaction with present occupation

Personal Data

Childhood emotional problems

Operations

Major illnesses
Bad accidents
Diseases
Smoking behavior—what and how much?
Drinking behavior—what and how much?
Narcotic drugs—which ones and how often?
Sleeping behavior
Suicide—attempted or considered
Chemical anesthetic—type(s)
Shock treatment—when and how many?

DIAGNOSTIC DATA

Conditioned Response Index. A 50-item test to determine the preparedness and level of suggestibility of a subject for hypnotherapy. The following coded behavioral traits are involved in the methodology of the CRI: Responsive—Analytical (RA); Cooperative—Resistant (CR); Concentration—Distractibility (CD); Imaginative—Unimaginative (IU); and Receptive—Suspicious (RS).

Correlational studies are conducted between test items, trait groups, and the total scores in relation to hypnotic induction methods, type of hypnotherapy and therapeutic results. The CRI was devised by Verdier (1965).

Ideomotor Response Questionnaire. Designed to get at the underlying causes of a disorder. It consists of 20 primary questions and a number of subquestions. See Appendix B for a copy of the questionnaire.

TREATMENT DATA

Visual imagery ability
Induction technique
   Progressive relaxation
   Arm levitation
   Repetitive movement
   Dynamic method
Maximum depth
   Hypnoidal
   Light
   Medium

Somnambulistic
Type of hypnotherapy employed
  Hypnoidal therapy
  Direct hypnotherapy
  Hypnoidal hypnoanalysis
  Reconstructive hypnoanalysis
Individual or group treatment
Treatment techniques used
Therapeutic time span (in months)
Number of sessions
Reason for termination
  Planned termination
  Withdrawal by client
Condition at termination
  Recovered
  Markedly improved
  Moderately improved
  Slightly improved
  Unimproved
  Worse

Evaluation Data

The following inventories are administered at the beginning and at the conclusion of therapy:

Fear Inventory. Seventy-six things and experiences that may cause fear. Each item is rated on a 5-point scale ranging from 'not at all' to 'very much.' This inventory was developed by Wolpe and Lazarus (1966).

Willoughby Schedule. A 25-item test for neuroticism relating mainly to common types of social situations. This questionnaire was developed by Willoughby (1932, 1934) and is a revision of the Thurstone Personality Schedule.

A I Questionnaire. A 30-item questionnaire intended to reveal specific areas of assertive and non-assertive interaction. This questionnaire was developed by Wolpe and Lazarus (1966).

Profile of Mood States (POMS). A 65-item adjective rating scale measuring the following dimensions of mood: Tension-Anxiety, Depression-Dejection, Anger-Hostility, Vigor-Activity, Fatigue-Inertia and Confusion-Bewilderment. In addition to the six factor scores, a Total Mood Disturbance Score may be obtained. This scale was developed by McNair, Lorr, and Droppleman (1971).

The Ego-strength Scale of the MMPI. Consists of 68 items from the Minnesota Multiphasic Personality Inventory. The scale was developed by Frank Barron (1953) for the purpose of predicting response to psychotherapy; it is interpreted as being essentially a measure of ego strength. The 68 items of the scale are arranged in the following groups: physical functioning and physiological stability, psychasthenia and seclusiveness, attitudes toward religion, moral posture, sense of reality, personal adequacy—ability to cope, phobias, miscellaneous.

FOLLOW-UP DATA

Symptoms and complaints for which client sought treatment are: same, better or worse.

Client's understanding of his or her condition: excellent, good, fair or poor.

Client's attitude toward therapist: friendly, indifferent or unfriendly.

A number of correlational studies have been conducted comparing all of the data presented in this chapter for every client.

Chapter 31.

A Structured Learning Approach to Training in Hypnotherapy

The training model to be presented here is an adaptation of the structured learning therapy model developed by Goldstein (1973).

Structured learning consists of four components, each of which is a well-established behavior change procedure. These procedures are modeling, role playing, social reinforcement and transfer training.

In each training session, a group of trainees (8 to 12) is:

(1) played a brief audiotape or videotape or shown a live presentation depicting a specific skill essential for the practice of professional hypnosis (modeling),

(2) given extensive opportunities to practice the skills they have learned (role playing),

(3) provided corrective feedback and approval as their role playing of the skill becomes more and more similar to the tape model's behavior (social reinforcement).

(4) Each of these procedures is carried out in such a way that transfer of the newly learned skills from the training setting to the trainee's professional setting will be highly likely (transfer training).

Structured learning modeling tapes are not instructional tapes in the usual sense. An instructional tape is most typically played to an audience that passively listens to it and then, at some later date, is supposed to do what was played. Such passive learning is not likely to be enduring learning. Thus, structured learning modeling tapes should not be played alone, i.e., without role playing and feedback following them. All four components of the structured learning training approach are necessary and sufficient for enduring learning of professional hypnosis skills.

The optimal size group for effective structured learning sessions consists of no more than 12 trainees. For both learning and transfer to occur, each trainee must have ample opportunity to practice what he has heard or seen modeled, receive feedback from the instructor and other trainees, and discuss his attempts to apply in his work setting what he has learned in the training sessions.

One basic skill portrayal is ideally covered in a two-hour training session. Approximately 1¼ hours are needed for the tape presentation-role playing-feedback sequence. The remaining time is spent in presentation and discussion of transfer attempts, i.e., homework.

The role-playing and feedback activities, which constitute most of each structured learning training session, are a series of "action-reaction" sequences in which effective skills are first rehearsed (role playing) and then critiqued (feedback). As such, the instructor must both lead and observe.

In addition to a need for proficiency in all aspects of clinical hypnosis, the hypnosis instructor who employs a structured learning approach to training must have proficiency in two additional types of skills. The first type of requisite skills are General Trainer Skills, i.e., those skills requisite for success in almost any training effort. These include flexibility and capacity for resourcefulness, listening skill, and group discussion leadership.

The second type of requisite skills are Specific Trainer Skills, i.e., those germane to structured learning in particular. These include an in-depth knowledge of structured learning, how to orient trainees to structured learning, how to initiate role playing, ability to present the material in a concrete, behavioral form, and procedures for providing corrective feedback.

All modeling tapes begin with the instructor setting the scene and stating the tape's learning points. Then the instructor portrays the skill to be learned. Each learning point is clearly enacted in sequence. The instructor then restates the learning points. This instructor introduction/modeling scene/instructor's summary constitutes the minimum requirement for a satisfactory modeling videotape or live structured learning presentation.

Of crucial importance is that the trainees seek to enact the learning points just modeled by the instructor. The learning points (steps in the particular procedure to be learned) should also be written on a chalkboard for the trainees to see while role playing. Trainees should take turns being the hypnotic operator and the subject. In addition, after modeling, but before role playing, each trainee should be given a card on which the learning points for the skill to be learned are typed or printed; these will be useful both during role playing as the hypnotic operator and when attempting to apply these points with an actual client. Before role playing begins, one trainee is selected to be the hypnotic operator and one is selected to be the hypnotic subject. The rest of the trainees are told to observe how well the trainee as hypnotic operator follows the learning points and to take notes on this for later discussion.

The role playing should continue until all trainees have had an opportunity to participate as hypnotic operator and subject. Upon completion of each role play, a brief feedback period should ensue. The goals of this activity are to let the trainee who was playing the role of hypnotic operator know how well he stayed with the learning points or in what ways he departed from them, and to provide him encouragement to try out his newly learned skills with an actual client. To implement this feedback process, the following sequence of eliciting comments has been found to be effective: comments from the trainee who role played the hypnotic subject, from the trainee who role played the hypnotic operator, from the observing trainees, and from the instructor who comments in particular on the following of the learning points and who provides positive reinforcement for close following.

In all critiques, it is crucial that the behavioral focus of structured learning be maintained. Comments must point to the presence or absence of specific, concrete points in regard to the skill to be learned, and not take form in general evaluative comments. Although feedback may be positive or negative in content, at minimum, a poor performance by the trainee operator can be praised as a "good try" at the same time that it is being criticized for its real faults. If at all possible, trainees failing to follow the relevant learning points in their role play should be given the opportunity to replay these same learning points after receiving corrective feedback. At times, we have videotaped entire role plays. Giving trainee operators later opportunities to observe themselves on tape can be an effective aid to learning.

As the final feedback step, after all role playing of the skill to be learned and discussion of it is completed, the modeling can be reenacted, or, if videotaped, the modeling tape can be replayed. This step summarizes the training session and leaves trainees with a final summary of the learning points.

Several aspects of the training sessions described above had as their prime purpose augmenting the likelihood that learning in the training setting will transfer to the trainee's actual real-life professional setting. Even more forthright steps should be taken to maximize transfer. A homework technique should be an integral part of any training program. In the structured learning homework procedure, trainees are instructed to try in their own professional settings the technique they have practiced during the session. The trainee is urged to take notes on his transfer attempts on a homework report form provided by the instructor, and, if possible, to tape each of his transfer attempts. The homework report form requests detailed information about what happened when the homework assignment was attempted and how well the relevant learning points were followed.

The Institute for Professional Hypnosis uses the structured learning approach to training in all of its classes. The class in clinical hypnosis and hypnotherapy (open only to psychotherapists, i.e., psychiatrists, clinical psychologists, psychiatric social workers or residents and interns in these fields), includes the teaching of skills pertaining to all of the phases of hypnotherapy. The following skills are taught in a step-by-step fashion: history taking, visual imagery training, hypnotic induction, deepening by the induction of graded responses, posthypnotic conditioning, training in self-hypnosis, the idea association technique, ideomotor questioning, the ego-strengthening technique, direct suggestions for symptom removal, attitude therapy by suggestion, hypnotic aversive conditioning, and how to achieve and test for the coma state.

The class in hypnoanalysis (also open only to psychotherapists) includes the teaching of the following skills that are taught to the client during the teaching phase of therapy prior to hypnoanalysis proper: posthypnotic amnesia, revivification, dreaming upon suggestion, positive hallucinations, and automatic writing. In addition, the following hypnoanalytic techniques are also taught in the hypnoanalysis course: directed association, techniques of graphic expression, techniques of plastic expression, hallucinatory techniques, hypnotic intensification of emotion and focusing techniques. The clinical hypnosis and hypnotherapy course is a prerequisite for the course in hypnoanalysis.

Each skill to be learned is broken down into individual steps. Good examples of the step-by-step procedure used in the structured learning approach to training are provided in Chapters 6, 9, 10, 16 and 18.

Recommended Reading

BOOKS

Ambrose, G. *Hypnotherapy with children.* London: Staples, 1961.

Arluck, E. *Hypnoanalysis: A case study.* New York: Random House, 1964.

Biddle, W. *Hypnosis and the psychoses.* Springfield, Ill.: Charles C. Thomas, 1967.

Brenman, M., and Gill, M. *Hypnotherapy.* New York: John Wiley, 1964. (Paperback edition)

Caprio, F., and Berger, J. *Helping yourself with self-hypnosis.* Englewood Cliffs, N. J.: Prentice-Hall, 1964.

Cheek, D., and LeCron, L. *Clinical hypnotherapy.* New York: Grune & Stratton, 1968.

Chertok, L. *Hypnosis.* New York: Pergamon Press, 1966.

Clement, P. *Hypnosis for therapists.* San Francisco, Calif.: Pierre Clement, publisher, 1970.

Crasilneck, H., and Hall, J. *Clinical hypnosis: Principles and application.* New York: Grune & Stratton, 1975.

Dengrove, E. *Hypnosis and behavior modification.* Springfield, Ill.: Charles C. Thomas, 1976.

Elman, D. *Findings in hypnosis.* Clifton, New Jersey: Author, 1964.

Erickson, M., Hershman, S., and Secter, I. *The practical applications of medical and dental hypnosis.* New York: Julian Press, 1961.

Freytag, F. *The hypnoanalysis of an anxiety hysteria.* New York: Julian Press, 1959.

Freytag, F. *Hypnosis and the body image.* New York: Julian Press, 1961.

Gill, M., and Brenman, M. *Hypnosis and related states.* New York: International Universities Press, 1959.

Gindes, B. *New concepts of hypnosis.* London: George Allen and Unwin, 1953.

Gordon, J. (Ed.) *Handbook of clinical and experimental hypnosis.* New York: Macmillan, 1966.

271

Haley, J. (Ed.) *Advanced techniques of hypnosis and therapy: Selected papers of Milton H. Erickson.* New York: Grune & Stratton, 1967.

Hartland, J. *Medical and dental hypnosis and its clinical applications.* Baltimore: Williams and Wilkins, 1966.

Hilgard, E. *Personality and hypnosis.* Chicago: University of Chicago Press, 1970.

Klemperer, E. *Past ego states emerging in hypnoanalysis.* Springfield, Ill.: Charles C. Thomas, 1968.

Kline, M. (Ed.) *Hypnodynamic psychology.* New York: Julian Press, 1955.

Kline, M. *Freud and hypnosis.* New York: The Institute for Research in Hypnosis Publication Society, 1958.

Kline, M. (Ed.) *Clinical correlations of experimental hypnosis.* Springfield, Ill.: Charles C. Thomas, 1963.

Kline, M. (Ed.) *Psychodynamics and hypnosis.* Springfield, Ill.: Charles C. Thomas, 1967.

Kroger, W. *Clinical and experimental hypnosis.* Philadelphia: Lippincott, 1963.

Kroger, W., and Fezler, W. *Hypnobehavioral therapy: Imagery conditioning.* Philadelphia: Lippincott, 1976.

LeCron, L. *Techniques of hypnotherapy.* New York: Julian Press, 1962.

LeCron, L. *Self hypnotism: The technique and its use in daily living.* Englewood Cliffs, N.J.: Prentice-Hall, 1964.

LeCron, L., and Bordeaux, J. *Hypnotism today.* New York: Grune & Stratton, 1947.

Lindner, R. *Rebel without a cause: The story of a criminal psychopath.* New York: Grove Press, 1944.

Marcuse, F. *Hypnosis: Fact and fiction.* Baltimore, Md.: Penguin Books, 1959.

Marcuse, F. (Ed.) *Hypnosis throughout the world.* Springfield, Ill.: Charles C. Thomas, 1964.

Meares, A. *Hypnography: A study in the therapeutic use of hypnotic painting.* Springfield, Ill.: Charles C. Thomas, 1957.

Meares, A. *Shapes of sanity: A study in the therapeutic use of modelling in the waking and hypnotic state.* Springfield, Ill.: Charles C. Thomas, 1960.

Meares, A. *A system of medical hypnosis.* Philadelphia: W. B. Saunders, 1960.

Moodie, W. *Hypnosis in treatment.* New York: Emerson Books, 1960.

Moss, C. *Hypnosis in perspective.* New York: Macmillan, 1965.

Rhodes, R. (Ed.) *Therapy through hypnosis.* New York: Citadel Press, 1952.

Rosen, H. *Hypnotherapy in clinical psychiatry.* New York: Julian Press, 1953.

Sacerdote, P. *Induced dreams.* New York: Vantage Press, 1967.

Schneck, J. *The principles and practice of hypnoanalysis.* Springfield, Ill.: Charles C. Thomas, 1965.

Van Pelt, S. *Modern hypnotism: Key to the mind.* Westport, Conn.: Associated Booksellers, 1956.

Van Pelt, S. *Secrets of hypnotism.* Hollywood, Calif.: Wilshire Book Co., 1958.

Weitzenhoffer, A. *General techniques of hypnotism.* New York: Grune & Stratton, 1957.

Wolberg, L. *Medical hypnosis.* New York: Grune & Stratton, 1948. (Two volumes.)

Wolberg, L. *Hypnoanalysis.* New York: Grune & Stratton, 1964. (2nd ed.)

JOURNALS

American Journal of Clinical Hypnosis.
Published by The American Society of Clinical Hypnosis.
Editorial Office: 401 Peachtree St. NE, Suite 804, Atlanta, Ga. 30308.

International Journal of Clinical and Experimental Hypnosis.
Published by The Society for Clinical and Experimental Hypnosis.
Editorial Office: 111 N. 49th St., Philadelphia, Pa. 19139.

The Journal of the American Institute of Hypnosis.
Published by the American Institute of Hypnosis.
Editorial Office: 7188 Sunset Blvd., Los Angeles, Calif. 90046.
No longer published. The last issue was in October, 1976 (Volume 17, No. 4).

Journal of the International Society for Professional Hypnosis.
Published by the International Society for Professional Hypnosis.
Editorial Office: 54 Willard Clark Circle, Spotswood, N.J. 08884.

British Journal of Clinical Hypnosis.
Published by the British Society of Medical and Dental Hypnosis.
Editorial Office: 14, Hawes Drive, Llandudno, Caernarvonshire, England.
No longer published. The last issue was in January, 1975 (Volume 5, No. 2).

British Journal of Medical Hypnotism.
Published by the British Society of Medical Hypnotists.
Editorial Office: 4, Victoria Terrace, Kingsway, Hove 3, Sussex, England.
No longer published. The last issue was the summer issue, 1966 (Volume 17, No. 4).

Appendix A

Historical Data Questionnaire

Date: _____

Examiner: _____

1. Name:
2. Age:
3. Birthplace:
4. Birth date:
5. Marital status:
6. Next of kin:
7. State in your own words your chief complaint:
8. How long has this been going on?
9. Was it a gradual or sudden onset?
10. Can you think of any reasons to explain this?
11. Whom have you previously consulted about your present problem?
12. What does your problem prevent you from doing?
13. What condition causes a variation in your illness?
    What seems to make it better?   What seems to make it worse?
14. Have you ever been hospitalized?
    If so, how many times and what for?
15. Do you have a history of recurrent illness appearing at certain
    times of the year or around times of emotional stress?
16. Have you had any major illnesses?
    If so, what and when?
17. Have you had any serious operations?
    If so, for what and when?
18. Have you been in any bad accidents?
    If so, what kind and when?
    What parts of the body were injured?
19. Have you lost any members of your family or any close friends
    through death? If so, state the relationship (i.e., mother, close
    friend, etc.) and how old you were at the time of death.
20. How did these experiences (numbers 14 through 19) affect you?

21. What diseases have you had (including childhood diseases)?
22. What was the best thing that ever happened to you?
23. What was the worst thing that ever happened to you?
24. What is your religious affiliation?
25. How often do you go to church?
26. Do you believe in the power of prayer?
27. What are your personal religious beliefs?
28. What place did religion play in your home life when you were growing up?
29. What is the earliest memory you can recall?
30. What is your earliest memory of your father?
31. What is your earliest memory of your mother?
32. Give a description of your father's personality and his attitude towards you (past and present):
33. Give a description of your mother's personality and her attitude towards you (past and present):
34. What were the dominant values and concerns of your family?
35. On looking back, do you feel that you owe more to your father or your mother?
36. Are you aware of having idealized and tried to be like one parent more than the other?
37. Did you feel more accepted and loved by one parent than the other? If so, which one?
38. Did you ever feel yourself to be a source of conflict between your parents?
39. How did your parents feel about each other?
40. Were there any especially difficult periods in their married life? If so, how old were you at the time and how did you feel about it?
41. In what way were you punished by your parents as a child?
42. Were you able to confide in your parents?
43. Has anyone (parents, relatives, friends, etc.) ever interfered in your choice of dates, occupation, friends, etc.?
44. Has any person within or outside of your family been of great influence in your life?
45. What kind of a person were you before your present problems developed?
46. Have you ever been in the military service? If so, what branch of service, what was your highest rank, where were you stationed, what were your duties and what were the dates of induction and discharge?
47. Do you have any nervous habits such as tics or nail-biting? If so, what nervous habits and what was the approximate date of onset?
48. Have you ever been arrested? If so, what for?   How many times?
49. Have you ever attempted suicide?

50. Have you ever thought about committing suicide?
51. Have you ever been given any form of chemical anesthetic? If so, please specify (i.e., ether).
52. Have you ever had shock treatments?
53. Have you ever used any narcotic drugs?
    If so, which ones and how often?
54. Do you smoke?
    If so, what (cigars, cigarettes, etc.) and how much?
55. Do you frequently have accidents?
56. Do you drink alcoholic beverages?
    If so, what and how often?
57. Do you sleep well?
58. What do you do with your spare time?
59. Do you make friends easily?
60. Are most of your friends of one sex? Which?
61. Can you confide in your friends?
62. What is your conception of a close friend?
63. What do you value in friends?
64. What is your present occupation?
65. How long have you been at it?
66. Are you happy at it?
67. Do you have any children?   If so, how many?   Ages?
68. How do they get along with each other?
69. Were you a healthy child?
70. Did you have any emotional problems as a child?
71. In general, how would you describe your childhood?
72. How did you get along in school?
73. What kind of grades did you make?
74. How far did you go in school (highest grade completed)?
75. How satisfied are you with your level of education?
76. What kinds of relationships did you establish with your teachers?
77. Did any of the following apply to you during childhood?

     (Circle ones that applied)

bed-wetting	sleep-walking
nail-biting	nightmares
thumb-sucking	running away
stealing	skipping school
stuttering	setting fires
temper tantrums	sexual confusion

     At what age or ages did each of the above occur and what was the frequency of each? (Enter after each circled item)

78. Did you date much in high school?
79. Did you have any difficulty getting along with the opposite sex?
80. What were your parents' attitudes towards sex?

81. Did you ever have any sexual conflicts or disturbing sexual experiences?
    If so, what were the conflicts or experiences and at what age or ages did they occur?
82. How old were you when you had your first sexual experience?
83. Have you ever had any homosexual relations?
84. (Ask if client is married): Have you had any extramarital relations?
85. Have you had any trouble with impotence (males) or frigidity (females)?
86. If married, how long have you been married?
87. Have you been married before?
    If so, tell how many times, length of each, and dates of each marriage or divorce.
88. How do you get along with your spouse?
89. What kind of a person is he (she)?
90. How does he (she) treat you?
91. Are you sexually satisfied in marriage?
92. Is your spouse?
93. What is your conception of the masculine role?
94. What is your conception of the feminine role?
95. Do you prefer to keep a certain distance from most other people?
96. Would you say that, by and large, you are a pessimist rather than an optimist?
97. Do you feel that, by and large, other people are to be trusted?
98. Who are the most important people in your life?
99. Does any member of your family suffer from alcoholism, drug addiction, or anything which could be considered a mental or emotional disorder?
100. Are there any other members of the family about whom information regarding illness, etc., is relevant?
101. Do you feel that you could benefit from hypnosis?
102. Why do you feel that hypnotic treatment would benefit you?
103. What do you think it feels like to be hypnotized?
104. If you wanted to relax yourself very deeply, or even to hypnotize yourself, how would you go about it (or what would you say to yourself)?
105. What actions were punished by your parents?
106. What actions were rewarded by your parents?
107. How many children were there in the family?
    (Give present ages and sex of each)
108. Please recount any fearful or distressing experiences not previously mentioned:
109. Is there anything that you haven't yet told me that you feel I really should know?

Appendix B

Hypnodiagnostic Association Test

Name:————————————————— Date:—————————

Age:————

Instructions to client (with client in hypnosis):

"I am going to call out a list of words and incomplete sentences to you. After I say each word, I want you to tell me the first word that comes into your mind after you hear my word. Likewise, when I give you an incomplete sentence, I would like you to complete the sentence, using the first thought that comes to mind. I want you to give me your response as quickly as you can. In case you are ever not certain what I have said, don't ask me to repeat it; but try to interpret it as well as you can and give me some response. I'll try to be clear so that you shouldn't have any trouble. Just say the first thing that comes into your mind in response to the word or incomplete sentence after you hear me say it."

Instructions to Therapist

This test allows the client to express his attitudes about many areas, including his feelings about hypnosis. Although there is no quantitative evaluation of test results, the following variables should be used for clinical interpretation: areas of rejection, indicated when there is a refusal to respond; areas of resistance, where there is a blocking or evasion by responding with a conventional or impersonal association; and other methods of evasion.

The following questions should be asked during the course of interpreting the test results: Are the client's responses stereotyped? Is he controlled or impulsive? Are his attitudes oriented in the direction of fantasy or are they basically realistic? Does the client respond primarily to drives from within himself or primarily from stimuli in the environment? Are his thought processes unsystematized or bizarre?

Although there is no quantitative evaluation of test results per se, the following broad scoring system may be utilized as a rough estimate of

Note.—The Institute for Professional Hypnosis
Copyright B. J. Hartman, 1976

the degree of conflict: (1) conflict, destructive or other unhealthy responses (assign a−); (2) positive, creative or healthy responses (assign a +); and (3) neutral or stereotyped responses (assign a 0). Responses falling into the minus category can be investigated further to determine the nature and degree of conflict.

Although a number of items could be grouped into categories such as sex, family and home, etc., it has been found more meaningful to treat each item separately. It has also been found that the client's responses are much more spontaneous and indicative of subconscious conflicts when the test is administered with the client in the hypnotic state.

1. Love _____
2. Father _____
3. Depressed _____
4. As a person, to myself, I am _____
5. As a person, to others, I am _____
6. Breast _____
7. Mother _____
8. Inside myself I am troubled _____
9. In my relationships with others I am troubled by _____

10. Problem _____
11. Fear _____
12. Life _____
13. When I feel badly, the feeling I most often have is _____

14. Death _____
15. If only _____
16. To be the person I want to be I must _____
17. I act as if I had no _____
18. Suicide _____
19. Why can't I _____
20. Mouth _____
21. I like _____
22. I am living as if I were _____
23. When the going gets too rough, I can always _____

24. House _____
25. Tongue _____
26. I feel happiest when _____
27. The future _____
28. Teeth _____
29. The one thing I need most is _____
30. My greatest fear is _____
31. People _____

32. Masturbate —————————————————————————
33. I secretly —————————————————————————
34. Doctor —————————————————————————
35. I need —————————————————————————
36. Please don't —————————————————————————
37. I'm sorry —————————————————————————
38. Marriage —————————————————————————
39. Hypnosis —————————————————————————
40. Man —————————————————————————
41. After death —————————————————————————
42. Underneath it all —————————————————————————
43. Penis —————————————————————————
44. Guilt —————————————————————————
45. Religion —————————————————————————
46. Ten years from now —————————————————————————
47. I lose control when —————————————————————————
48. Hostility —————————————————————————
49. I failed —————————————————————————
50. I resent —————————————————————————
51. When I was younger —————————————————————————
52. Vagina —————————————————————————
53. Escape —————————————————————————
54. I feel sad when —————————————————————————
55. Compared with others, I —————————————————————————
56. Affection —————————————————————————
57. Hospital —————————————————————————
58. Woman —————————————————————————
59. I'm just tired of —————————————————————————
60. I think of myself as —————————————————————————
61. Freedom —————————————————————————
62. Authority —————————————————————————
63. I dislike to —————————————————————————
64. Trust —————————————————————————
65. Operation —————————————————————————
66. I'll be OK when —————————————————————————
67. If I were King (or Queen), I would —————————————————————————
68. Confinement —————————————————————————
69. When I'm on top —————————————————————————
70. It's so easy to —————————————————————————
71. My deepest thoughts tell me —————————————————————————
72. Relax —————————————————————————
73. Birth —————————————————————————
74. When others rely on me, I —————————————————————————
75. My sexual desires —————————————————————————
76. People who give orders —————————————————————————

77. What I want most from hypnosis is ⸺⸺⸺⸺
78. Responsibility ⸺⸺⸺⸺⸺⸺⸺
79. Most of all I want ⸺⸺⸺⸺⸺⸺
80. I believe in ⸺⸺⸺⸺⸺⸺⸺
81. When I disobeyed my father ⸺⸺⸺⸺
82. When I have to make a decision, I ⸺⸺⸺
83. Sexual intercourse ⸺⸺⸺⸺⸺
84. It's so easy to ⸺⸺⸺⸺⸺⸺
85. My family ⸺⸺⸺⸺⸺⸺⸺
86. I enjoy ⸺⸺⸺⸺⸺⸺⸺⸺
87. If I had one wish, I would ⸺⸺⸺⸺
88. Hypnosis can best help me by ⸺⸺⸺⸺
89. The thing I remember best about childhood is ⸺⸺
90. The core of my identity is ⸺⸺⸺⸺
91. Never call me ⸺⸺⸺⸺⸺⸺
92. My best asset is ⸺⸺⸺⸺⸺⸺
93. I can't ⸺⸺⸺⸺⸺⸺⸺⸺
94. I experience conflict when I ⸺⸺⸺⸺
95. The change I intend to accomplish in therapy is ⸺⸺

Appendix C

Ideomotor Response Questionnaire

Name:—————————————————— Date:——————————

Age:————

Instructions to client (with client in hypnosis):

"The causes of emotional problems vary greatly. The true cause or causes for your problem are known only by your subconscious mind. If you knew consciously what the causes were for your problem, you wouldn't be here. Therefore, I am going to ask your subconscious mind some questions, and the answers will help us to get to the heart of your problem. In hypnosis, we are able to communicate directly with your subconscious mind. Your subconscious mind is like a tape recorder; it is a storehouse of every experience, memory or thought you have had since you were born.

"When I ask the questions, your subconscious mind will reply by lifting the right forefinger (touch designated finger of subject) to indicate yes; the left forefinger to indicate no; the right thumb to indicate 'I don't know'; and the left thumb to indicate 'I don't want to answer'. These two fingers and thumbs (touch them) are now under the control of your subconscious mind. They will respond to my questions without any deliberate thought or control on your part. There is nothing mysterious about this. Your subconscious mind controls all of the autonomic or involuntary functions of your body, such as breathing, heartbeat and regulation of body temperature. All of the functions of the autonomic nervous system, which are involuntary in the normal waking state, can be controlled in hypnosis because the subconscious mind, which controls these involuntary functions, can be communicated with directly.

———————————————

Note.—The National Foundation for Research in Clinical Hypnosis

"And now I want you to imagine, to visualize, the most relaxed and pleasant scene imaginable. Visualize any scene that is comfortable. It can be nothing more than being at a beach watching the water break on the shore. Or a lake with a sailboat floating lazily by. Any scene that is pleasant and makes you feel good. Become part of that scene, experience everything about it and enjoy it completely. In a moment I am going to begin asking questions. I want you to continue visualizing and enjoying the pleasant scene. I don't want you to exert any conscious effort to hear the questions I am asking because I will be talking to your subconscious mind, and in order to get a true subconscious answer, the less conscious interference, the better. Just continue enjoying your scene, and in a moment I will begin communication with your subconscious mind."

Instructions to therapist

After determining the nature of the "key" to the illness or symptom, proceed to discover:

1. The number of repetitions of the key causal factor
2. Their order of importance for the subconscious mind
3. The order in which they should be dealt with

Questions

1. Do you want to understand the meaning of your symptom?
2. I want to know if you really want help with this problem, whether you really want to give up your symptom?
3. Is it all right for you to know the causes of (name symptom)?
4. Is there some underlying motivation for your symptom?
   (If answer is affirmative, ask the following:)
   Is this motive serving to protect you in some way or to defend you against something?
   Is it getting you out of something?
   Are you seeking sympathy and attention with your symptom?
   Is it preventing you from doing something?
   Is it serving some other purpose?
5. Are you identifying with someone else as a cause of your condition —trying to be like someone else?
   (If affirmative, ask the following:)
   Is it your mother?
   Is it your father?
   Is it some other relative?
   (brother, sister, aunt, uncle, grandparent, etc.)
   Is it someone else?
   (friend, teacher, etc.)
6. We can feel guilty about things we do, even about thoughts we may have. Is this a punishment for something? Are you punishing yourself for some reason?

(If affirmative, ask the following:)

Do you feel guilty about something?

Is it about something definite rather than for ideas or general guilt feelings?

The (name symptom) began about (specify time of onset). Possibly you felt guilty about something that happened a long time ago, or it might have been just before the onset of your condition. Was it something recent, within the past two years?

Was it within a short time before (name symptom) began?

Did you do something you considered sexually immoral? (cover other major areas, i.e., dishonesty, disloyalty, etc.)

7. Is your problem related to or connected with some experience of your past?

(If affirmative, ask the following:)

Is there more than one incident?

We should learn when this experience took place.

Was it something that occurred before you were (start several years before present age and keep going back until age of experience is pinpointed).

Was it concerned with an illness?

Was it concerned with an operation?

Was it concerned with an accident?

Was it concerned with the death of someone close to you?

Did it happen indoors rather than outdoors?

Was any other person involved?

Were you hurt at the time?

Go back to that time and place and let your "yes" finger rise up to indicate when you are there. As your finger lifts, the event will come clearly into your mind and you can speak about it if you feel it is all right.

8. Has someone ever said anything to you that has something to do with causing your present condition? Is there a suggestion of any kind being carried out?

(If affirmative, ask the following:)

Is there more than one suggestion being carried out?

We should learn when this suggestion was given to you. Was it before you were (start several years before present age and keep going back until age when the suggestion was given is pinpointed).

Was it concerned with an illness or an operation?

Was it concerned with an accident?

Was the suggestion given to you at home? at school? at a friend's home? at church? at a doctor or dentist's office? in a hospital?

Was the suggestion given to you by (use location as a lead, i.e., at home—mother, father, etc.; at school—teacher).

(Instruct subject to go back to that time and place and let his "yes" finger rise up to indicate when he is there. Then tell subject,

"As your finger lifts, the suggestion will come clearly into your mind.")

9. Is there an underlying conflict connected with your problem?
(If affirmative, ask the following:)
Is it a conflict concerning sex?
Is it a conflict concerning dependency vs. independence?
Is it a conflict concerning feelings of love and hate?
Is it concerned with your parents?
Is it concerned with your spouse or your children?
Is it concerned with your religious beliefs?

10. Is there anything or anyone in your present environment causing or contributing to your problem?
(If affirmative, name all possible things and people until you have pinpointed the environmental causes.)

11. (Ask this question only if some physical symptomotology is involved. This question is designed to ascertain whether organ language is involved.)
Do you have this (name symptom, i.e., headache) because something or someone is a (headache, pain in the neck, etc.) to you?

12. Are you holding on to your symptom out of spite?
Are you using your symptom to get back at someone for some reason?
(If affirmative, ask the following:)
Is it your mother?
It is your father?
Is it some other relative?
    (brother, sister, aunt, uncle, grandparent, etc.)
Is it someone else?
    (friend, teacher, etc.)

13. Are you holding on to your symptom because you are afraid to grow up?

14. Is your problem related to or connected with a wish for failure?

15. Is your problem related to or connected with a fear of success?

16. Does your symptom in any way serve as a replacement of a lost object?

17. Are there past conditionings present as a cause of your condition?
(If affirmative, ask the following:)
Are family beliefs responsible for your problem?
Are local standards responsible?
Are caste and/or religious restrictions responsible?
Are educationally imposed beliefs responsible?

18. Is there any other reason for this condition other than (name the ones already discovered)?

19. Now that you understand the true causes of your condition, can you now be free of (name symptom)?

20. Do you feel that any further treatment is necessary at this time in order to remain free of (name symptom)?

Glossary

The student in clinical hypnosis is confronted with numerous terms in the professional journals and textbooks which are not defined for him and which are either not included in standard dictionaries or, if included, are often inadequately defined. The need for an up-to-date glossary covering all of the words used in every aspect of hypnosis has been apparent for many years. I feel that this glossary adequately satisfies that need.

ABREACTION. A mental process in which forgotten memories are relived with a display of appropriate emotions.

AFFECT. Any experience of emotion or feeling.

AGE PROGRESSION. A pseudoorientation in time whereby an individual is taken into the future while in hypnosis.

AGE REGRESSION. A hypnotic phenomenon of returning to an earlier period of life.

AMNESIA. A partial or complete inability to recall or identify past experiences. Loss of memory.

AMNESIA, ANTEROGRADE. A loss of memory for events following trauma or shock.

AMNESIA, AUTOHYPNOTIC. A self-induced repression of certain memories.

AMNESIA, RETROGRADE. An inability to remember experiences extending backward in time from the onset of amnesia.

AMNESIA, SPONTANEOUS. A form of amnesia occurring in a subject without any suggestion to this effect.

ANALGESIA. An absence of sensibility to pain.

ANAMNESIS. A developmental history of an individual and of his illness, especially a patient's recollections.

ANESTHESIA. An absence of feeling. It may be local or general, total or partial.

ANIMAL MAGNETISM. Anton Mesmer's term for hypnosis, based on the incorrect notion that the phenomena observed were due to the emanation of a magnetic fluid or force.

ARTIFICIAL DREAM. A voluntarily invented plot imitating the contents of a dream.

ASSOCIATION. An expression of ideas or words of which one thinks in connection with an experience. (See also FREE ASSOCIATION.)

ATAVISM. A reversion to the characteristics of a remote ancestor.

ATONICITY. A lack of normal muscle tone.

AUDITORY HALLUCINATION. Auditory perception without an appropriate external stimulus.

AUTISTIC THINKING. Imaginary gratification of desires in fantasy as contrasted with realistic attempts to gratify them.

AUTOANALYSIS. Self-analysis.

AUTOCONDITIONING. A form of self-hypnosis developed by Dr. Hornell Hart.

AUTOGENIC TRAINING. A graduated series of mental exercises designed to produce a general psychobiologic reorganization. The resultant changes improve the individual's capacity for introspection and purposeful activity. Developed in Germany by Dr. Schultz approximately 50 years ago. Schultz trained patients to go into self-induced hypnosislike states.

AUTOHYPNOSIS. A kind of verbal conditioning whereby the hypnotic state is induced by the subject himself and he alone retains control of what is to follow.

AUTOMATIC DRAWING. Drawing without conscious control. This is a technique used in hypnoanalysis.

AUTOMATIC SPEECH. Verbalizations uttered in a state of mental dissociation, without the aid of conscious awareness.

AUTOMATIC WRITING. Writing without conscious control. Automatic activity of the hand while the subject's attention is directed elsewhere. A technique used in hypnoanalysis.

AUTOMATISM. Any activity performed without the conscious awareness of the individual, or in which the normal exercise of the will is in abeyance.

AUTONOMIC NERVOUS SYSTEM. The section of the nervous system that regulates the internal organs. It consists primarily of ganglia connected with the brain stem and spinal cord and may be subdivided into the sympathetic and parasympathetic systems.

AUTOSUGGESTION. A suggestion that emanates from the individual himself.

BAQUET. A large tub used by Mesmer for his hypnotic seances. The tub was filled with water and iron filings, and patients would stand around the tub and touch iron rods protruding from the water. A contact with the rods was thought to originate magnetic currents.

BIBLIOTHERAPY. The use of reading as an adjunctive aid in the psychotherapeutic treatment of psychological disorders.

BLOCKING. An involuntary inhibition of recall, ideation, or communication, including sudden stoppage of speech.

BODY IMAGE. The mental image one has of one's body.

BRAIN WAVES. Minute electrical oscillations given off by the cerebral cortex.

BRAIN WAVE SYNCHRONIZER. An electrical instrument designed to induce various levels of hypnosis by photic stimulation of the brain waves.

CATALEPSY. A condition of muscular rigidity in which the limbs or body remain passively in any position in which they are placed.

CATHARSIS. A discharge of emotional tension associated with repressed traumatic material by "talking it out."

CATHEXIS. An emotional charge. The concentration of psychic energy on an idea or object.

CLONUS. Rapid, oscillatory movements in which muscular rigidity and relaxation rapidly follow each other.

CLOUDED CONSCIOUSNESS. Disorientation and unclear perception due to sensory disturbance.

COLLECTIVE UNCONSCIOUS. In Jungian theory, a portion of the unconscious common to all mankind; also called RACIAL UNCONSCIOUS.

COMA. A stupor of such depth that all consciousness is gone.

CONCENTRATED ATTENTION, LAW OF. The principle that states that whenever attention is concentrated on an idea over and over again, it spontaneously tends to realize itself.

CONDENSATION. A telescoping of images in a dream. This process transfers the affect from a group of ideas to one idea.

CONDITIONED REFLEX. An induced reflex developed by repetitive experience in association with another stimulus.

CONSCIOUSNESS. The state of being aware; that part of the mind which is aware of phenomena taking place inside and outside of the personality.

CONVERSION. A symbolic expression of psychological conflict in motor or sensory symptoms.

CORTICAL FREQUENCY SPECTRUM. A range of electrical waves produced by the brain.

COUNTERSUGGESTION. A suggestion offered to an individual to challenge his belief concerning something.

COUNTERTRANSFERENCE. A therapist's conscious or unconscious emotional reaction to his patient.

CRYPTOMNESIA. A spontaneous recall of events or items of knowledge without being able to recall the circumstances or time when the knowledge was originally gained.

DAYDREAMING. Reverie. Free play of thought or imagination.

DEFENSE MECHANISM. Any of several specific intrapsychic defensive processes, operating unconsciously, which are employed to seek resolution of emotional conflict and freedom from anxiety.

DEHYPNOTIZATION. Bringing a subject out of hypnosis.

DELUSION. A belief contrary to reality and held in spite of evidence and common sense.

DEPERSONALIZATION. A loss of the sense of personal identity; or a sensation of having no material existence.

DEPTH PSYCHOLOGY. The psychology of unconscious mental processes.

DEPTH REVERSAL. In hypnosis, refers to reversing the depth of the hypnotic state, such as bringing the subject from a deeper to a lighter stage.

DEPTH SCORE. The depth or profundity of a trance as measured by a scale of hypnotic susceptibility.

DESENSITIZATION. Removing a complex or rendering it less disturbing. This is a therapeutic process by means of which reactions to traumatic experiences are reduced in intensity by repeatedly exposing the individual to them in mild form, either in reality or fantasy.

DIAGNOSIS. A recognition and identification of a disease or specific problem.

DISORIENTATION. A loss of awareness of the position of the self in relation to place, time, or person.

DISSOCIATION. A psychologic separation or splitting off. An intrapsychic defensive process which operates automatically and unconsciously. The separated part of the personality functions as another whole, as though it represented another person.

DISTORTION. In psychoanalytic theory, a mechanism which, in dreams, together with condensation, symbolization and overdetermination, aids in the repression and disguise of unacceptable thoughts.

DOMINANT EFFECT, LAW OF. A law based on the axiom that a strong emotion tends to replace a weaker one. Also, attaching a strong emotion to a suggestion tends to make the suggestion more effective.

DREAM. A train of hallucinatory experiences with a certain degree of coherence, but often confused and bizarre, taking place during sleep and in similar conditions.

DRUG HYPNOSIS. The use of drugs in conjunction with hypnosis. (See NARCOTHERAPY.)

EEG. Electroencephalogram. The recording of brain waves.

EIDETIC IMAGE. An unusually vivid and apparently exact mental image. It may be a memory, fantasy, or dream.

ELABORATION. An unconscious psychologic process of expansion and elaboration of detail, especially with reference to a symbol or repesentation in a dream.

ELECTRONARCOSIS. Electrically induced sleep.

EUPHORIA. An exaggerated feeling of physical and emotional well-being, usually of psychologic origin. In its nontechnical sense, it also connotes contentment or happiness.

FACILITATION. In hypnosis, the increased ease of performing certain bodily activities as a result of hypnotic suggestion.

FANTASY. Forming mental images of scenes, often in sequences, of experiences that have not actually happened or that have happened in a way considerably different from that fantasied.

FIXATION. In hypnosis, the directing and focussing of both eyes on an object or point.

FLACCIDITY. A state of limpness, without normal tonus, and therefore easily giving way to pressure.

FORECONSCIOUS. Preconscious. Material not ordinarily in consciousness but subject to voluntary recall.

FREE ASSOCIATION. Saying whatever comes to mind; a basic rule in psychoanalysis.

FUNCTIONAL DISORDER. A disorder of emotional origin in which organic or structural changes are either absent or are developed secondarily to prolonged emotional stress.

GLOVE ANESTHESIA. Anesthesia of the hand; sometimes a hysterical symptom but can also be produced in hypnosis.

GRADING. Suggestions are graded according to the ease of acceptance. In inducing hypnosis, the patient is first given suggestions which are easy to accept and then suggestions which are progressively more difficult.

GROUP HYPNOSIS. Hypnotic conditioning or hypnotherapy conducted with more than one patient at a time.

HALLUCINATED UNCONSCIOUS BODY IMAGE. A picture that an individual unconsciously forms of himself in his own unconscious mind. This projective technique and psychotherapeutic approach is made achievable by the use of hypnosis and has been extensively investigated by Dr. Fredericka Freytag.

HALLUCINATION. A false sensory perception in the absence of an actual external stimulus; may be emotional or chemical (drugs, etc.) origin and may occur in any of the five senses.

HEMI-HYPNOSIS. A hypnotic state in which voluntary activities are confined to one side of the body as a result of hypnotic suggestion.

HETEROACTION. The effect whenever the response to a suggestion alters the response to a subsequent but different suggestion.

HETEROHYPNOSIS. The process of inducing the hypnotic state in another person.

HETEROSUGGESTION. A suggestion given by an individual to another person.

HISTRIONIC. Pertaining to dramatic representation.

HOMOACTION. The effect whenever the response to a suggestion alters the response to a subsequent repetition of this suggestion.

HYPERACUITY. An unusual degree of sensitiveness of sight, hearing, touch, smell or taste due to psychological causes alone.

HYPERACUSIA. Abnormal keenness of hearing.

HYPERAESTHESIA. An unusal degree of sensitivity of the actual sense organs.

HYPERALGESIA. An excessive sensitivity to pain.

HYPERAPHIA. An abnormal sensitivity of the sense of touch.

HYPERKINESIS. An excessive muscular action.

HYPERMNESIA. An unusal ability to recall or remember past experiences.

HYPERPNEA. Very rapid breathing; sometimes a hysterical symptom.

HYPERPRAXIA. An unusual increase of muscular power.

HYPERPROSEXIA. An extreme concentration of attention on a part of the field of observation to the exclusion of everything else.

HYPERSOMNIA. A morbid condition in which the patient sleeps for an excessively long time and is given to drowsiness.

HYPERTHYMIA. An exaggerated emotional excitement.

HYPERTONICITY. An increased muscle tonus accompanied by increased excitability of reflexes, especially those involving antigravity muscles.

HYPNAGOGIC THOUGHT. A flash of thought perceived in the semiconscious state leading into the state of sleep.

HYPNOAID. Any device that aids the operator in hypnotic induction.

HYPNODELIC. Refers to the combined use of hypnosis and LSD in conjunction with psychotherapy.

HYPNODIAGNOSIS. Identifying a disorder with the aid of hypnosis.

HYPNODISC. A spiral disc, either revolving or nonrevolving, which serves the purpose of eye fixation and eye fatigue; used as an aid for hypnotic induction.

HYPNODRAMA. The application of psychodrama techniques in conjunction with hypnosis.

HYPNOGENIC. Sleep-producing. Inducing hypnosis or trance states by methods that first bring about drowsiness or sleep.

HYPNOGRAPHOLOGY. A technique in hypnoanalysis in which the handwriting of the hypnotized patient is analyzed, either at his present age or at various ages in the past.

HYPNOGRAPHY. A technique in hypnoanalysis in which the hypnotized patient projects psychic material in black and white painting.

HYPNOIDAL. A stage before that of hypnosis. Characterized by some detachment as well as by physical relaxation and heightened suggestibility.

HYPNOLOGY. A term used by Braid for the study and practice of hypnosis. Also refers to the scientific investigation of sleep.

HYPNOMNEMONICS. The use of natural sleep, artificial sleep, or of hypnosis as an aid to memorizing and/or recalling.

HYPNONARCOSIS. Hypnotherapy conducted under the influence of narcotic drugs.

HYPNOPEDIA. Teaching in hypnotic trance by means of a tape recorder.

HYPNOPLASTY. A technique in hypnoanalysis in which the patient uses clay to model whatever he wishes to make. The patient is asked to associate to the model and the disclosed material is used in his hypnoanalytic handling.

HYPNOSEMANTICS. The investigation of the meaning of words used in hypnotic induction.

HYPNOSIS. An induced psychological state characterized by increased suggestibility, concentration, physical and mental relaxation, selective inattention, heightened ability for fantasy production, a reduction in reality testing and a tolerance for reality distortion. This state results in the facilitation or inhibition of muscular response, changes in sensory thresholds and the improvement of recall, which may be induced more readily than in the normal waking state and may be effected either by the individual himself or by another person known as the hypnotic operator.

HYPNOSLEEP. Hypnosis attached to sleep; bringing on the hypnotic state during sleep. This is the deepest stage of hypnosis.

HYPNOTARIUM. A special room, slightly darkened, used for hypnotic treatment. This term appeared in the Russian literature.

HYPNOTIC. Relating to hypnosis. Also, drug producing hypnosis or sleep.

HYPNOTIC ABLATION. A technique consisting of having the hypnotized subject regress to an earlier age.

HYPNOTIC DREAM. A dream produced through direct or indirect posthypnotic suggestion.

HYPNOTISM. The scientific study and practice of hypnosis.

HYPNOTIZABILITY. The capacity of an individual to be hypnotized.

HYPOFUNCTION. A lowered functioning or activity of an organ.

HYPOKINESIS. A lowered vigor of movement or motor response.

HYPOTAXY. A phase of hypnotism that prepares the organism to be responsive to suggestions.

IATROGENIC ILLNESS. An emotional illness unwittingly precipitated by the physician's attitude, examination, or comments.

IATROPSYCHOLOGY. The application of psychological concepts in medical practice. Its influence shows in the current focus of attention on psychosomatics. Dr. Jerome Schneck coined the term.

IDEA OF INFLUENCE. A false belief that one's thoughts are being influenced by some outside agency, such as hypnosis.

IDEAS OF REFERENCE. An incorrect interpretation of casual incidents and external events as having direct reference to oneself. May reach sufficient intensity to constitute delusions.

IDEOMOTOR ACTIVITY. The involuntary capacity of muscles to respond instantaneously to thoughts, feelings and ideas.

IDEOPLASTY. A process whereby the subject's mind is made receptive by means of useful suggestions given by the hypnotic operator.

IDEOSENSORY ACTIVITY. The capacity of the brain to develop sensory images, which may be kinesthetic, olfactory, visual, auditory, tactile or gustatory.

ILLUSION. A false interpretation of an actual perception.

IMAGERY. A collective term for mental images. It may pertain to any of the five senses, although it usually refers to those of vision or hearing.

IMAGINATION. Mentally shaping and synthesizing objects or ideas into pictures or patterns different from any involved in one's previous experience.

INDUCED HALLUCINATION. A hallucination produced as the result of hypnotic suggestion.

INDUCTION. In hypnosis, the act of inducing a hypnotic state.

INNERVATION. A nervous excitation or stimulation of a muscle or other organ.

INSIGHT. Self-understanding. The extent of the original, nature and mechanisms of an individual's attitudes and behavior.

INSIGHT THERAPY. A treatment which strives to show the patient his underlying conflicts with the purpose of effecting a change in his personality.

INTRAPSYCHIC. That which takes place within the psyche or mind.

INTROSPECTION. Looking into oneself. Preoccupation with one's thoughts and feelings.

INTUITION. Instant knowledge obtained without reasoning. A popular rather than scientific term.

INVOLUNTARY. Referring to an action taking place independently of an individual's will, but not necessarily in spite of it.

JAPANESE ILLUSION. A confusion of the sense of touch caused by the intertwining of the fingers.

KINESTHETIC. The sense pertaining to muscular movement.

KOHNSTAMM TEST. A test often used to demonstrate suggestibility to a subject being prepared for hypnosis. It is a normal neuro-physiologic reaction, elicited by having the subject press his extended arm as strenuously as possible against a wall for several minutes, after which the arm will rise automatically with or without a suggestion to that effect.

LATENT CONTENT. The deeper symbolic level of a dream. Repressed wishes that are indirectly expressed in the manifest content of dreams.

LETHARGY. Drowsiness, inaction and apathy.

LIBIDO. Constructive or destructive psychic energy.

MANIFEST CONTENT. The content of a dream as the dreamer remembers it.

MESMERISM. Animal magnetism. Obsolete term for hypnotism.

METRONOME. An instrument for indicating and marking exact time in music, consisting usually of a reversed pendulum whose period of vibration is regulated by a shifting weight. Metronomes are sometimes used as an aid to hypnotic induction.

MONOIDEISM. A term coined by Dr. James Braid to refer to the hypnotic state. He had coined the term *hypnosis* but when he discovered that hypnosis is not related to sleep, he felt that the term *monoideism* more accurately described the hypnotic state.

MULTIPLE PERSONALITY. A type of dissociative reaction charac-terized by two or more relatively independent personality systems in the same individual.

MUSCLE READING. The art of inferring the thoughts of a person in simple situations through his involuntary muscular movements.

NANCY SCHOOL. The hypnotic school of thought headed by Drs. Liebeault and Bernheim. This school held that hypnosis is a form of suggestion. For a number of years, a controversy raged between the Nancy School and the Salpetriere or Paris School headed by Dr. Charcot. The Nancy School triumphed over the views of Charcot.

NARCOHYPNOANALYSIS. The use of drugs in conjunction with hypnoanalysis.

NARCOLEPSY. Brief, uncontrollable episodes of sleeping.

NARCOSIS. A deep unconsciousness induced by a narcotic drug.

NARCOSYNTHESIS. A treatment technique in which hypnotic drugs are used for releasing the patient's inhibitions to reveal intimate information. The discharged emotional material is collected and synthesized by doctor and patient.

NARCOTHERAPY. The use of drugs to facilitate the release of un-conscious material.

NEGATIVE HALLUCINATION. An absence of a sense experience in the presence of appropriate sensory stimuli.

NEGATIVE TRANSFERENCE. Hostile and antagonistic feelings that the patient develops toward the therapist or that the therapist develops toward the patient.

NEUROSIS. A functional personality disorder in which there is no gross personality disorganization and for which the patient does not ordinarily require hospitalization; synonymous with psychoneurotic disorder.

NEURYPNOLOGY. Nervous sleep. Braid's original term to describe hypnosis. Also, the title of Braid's book published in 1843.

OBJECT RELATIONSHIP. The quality of the relationship between the individual and people and things in his environment.

OLFACTORY HALLUCINATION. Smelling something that is not present and that no odor present suggests.

ONEIROLOGY. The science concerned with the study of dreams.

ORGANIC DISORDER. Characterized by demonstrable structural or biochemical changes in the tissues and organs of the body as distinguished from an emotional disorder.

ORIENTATON. An awareness of oneself in relation to time, place, and person.

PARESTHESIA. Abnormal, distorted, or wrongly localized sensation.

PARALYSIS, HYPNOTIC. A temporary loss of motor functioning in some part of the body as a result of hypnotic suggestion.

PARAMNESIA. False memory. Distorted recollection or memory of some past event. It may refer to inclusion of false details, omission of details, or distortion of time references.

PARASYMPATHETIC DIVISION. A division of the autonomic nervous system. It is active in relaxed or quiescent states of the body and to some extent antagonistic to the sympathetic division. (See SYMPATHETIC DIVISION.)

PARIS SCHOOL. The hypnotic school of thought headed by Charcot. This school held that hypnotic phenomena were related to hysteria.

PASSES. Refers to sweeping motions over the subject's body. Passes, with or without bodily contact, were frequently used by early pioneers in hypnosis and were thought to be helpful in hypnotic induction.

PERCEPTON. Awareness of a stimulus.

PERSEVERATION. The tendency of an idea, feeling, or mode of activity to recur after the original experience.

PERSONAL UNCONSCIOUS. The part of the unconscious that develops as a result of individual experience.

PHOTIC ACTIVATION. A technique for exaggerating the EEG by light stimulation.

PHRENOMAGNETISM. An outmoded approach to hypnotic induction. It involves invoking a trance directly by pressing a skull protuberance.

PLACEBO. An inactive substance administered in place of an active drug.

PLANCHETTE. A heart-shaped board supported by two legs, used for obtaining automatic writing.

PLASTOTHERAPY. A method of using clay modeling as a vehicle for psychotherapy; free association to the clay model.

POSITIVE HALLUCINATION. A hypnotic phenomenon of having a sense experience in the absence of appropriate sensory stimuli.

POSTHYPNOTIC AMNESIA. A state of amnesia that occurs upon awakening from hypnosis, for events that took place during the hypnotic state. It is usually the result of a posthypnotic suggestion, but it also may occur spontaneously.

POSTHYPNOTIC SUGGESTION. A suggestion given in hypnosis that the subject later executes in the waking state. He usually does so without recalling the suggestion originally given him.

PRECONSCIOUS. Refers to thoughts that are not in immediate awareness, but that can be recalled by conscious effort.

PREHYPNOTIC SUGGESTION. A suggestion given to the subject before going into hypnosis.

PROJECTION. A mental mechanism whereby that which is emotionally unacceptable in the self is unconsciously rejected and attributed to others.

PROJECTIVE HYPNOANALYSIS. An hypnoanalytic technique utilizing the combined tactics of psychoanalysis, hypnosis, and projective techniques. It makes use of free association, dream analysis, and transference reactions as they are projected onto relatively unstructured situations in hypnosis.

PROJECTIVE TEST. A personality test based upon responses to relatively unstructured materials and situations.

PSYCHOCYBERNETICS. The conception of the human brain and nervous system as a form of servomechanism, operating in accordance with cybernetic principles. The principles of cybernetics as applied to the human brain.

PSYCHOGENIC. Of mental origin; originating in the psychological functioning of the individual.

PSYCHOMOTOR. Involving both psychological and physical activity.

PSYCHOMOTOR EXCITEMENT. A generalized physical and emotional overactivity in response to internal and/or external stimuli.

PSYCHOMOTOR RETARDATION. A generalized retardation of physical and emotional reactions.

PSYCHONEUROSIS. Neurosis.

PSYCHOPATHOLOGY. The field of science dealing with the causes and nature of abnormal behavior.

PSYCHOPHARMACOLOGY. An interdisciplinary science that is concerned with the study of the effects of drugs on behavior.

PSYCHOPHYSIOLOGIC DISORDER. Physical symptoms resulting from the continued emotional mobilization during sustained stress. Often involves actual tissue damage.

PSYCHOSIS. A severe personality disorder involving loss of contact with reality and usually characterized by delusions and hallucinations.

RAPPORT. An interpersonal relationship characterized by mutual con-operation, confidence, and harmony.

RECALL. In hypnosis, refers to the remembering of events which have been consciously forgotton. The form of remembering in which the subject demonstrates retention by repeating what was earlier learned.

RECIPROCAL INHIBITION. The relationship between muscles that are controlled through reciprocal innervation.

RECIPROCAL INNERVATION. A form of neural integration in which one of a pair of antagonistic muscles is actively inhibited when the other member of the pair contracts.

RECONSTRUCTIVE PSYCHOTHERAPY. A psychological treatment directed toward a fundamental reorganization of the basic personality structure and dynamics of the patient.

REVERIE. More or less aimless trains of imagery and ideas, often of the nature of daydreaming.

REVIVIFICATION. In hypnosis, when the subject actualy relives earlier events of his life. All memories following the age to which the subject is regressed are ablated.

SCENE VISUALIZATION. Refers to the mental pictures produced in hypnosis. A hypnotherapeutic technique.

SCREEN MEMORY. A true memory that is used to hide another memory of a related experience.

SENSITIVITY. Susceptibility to stimulation. Ability to be affected by, and respond to, stimuli of low intensity, or to slight stimulus differences.

SENSORIUM. Includes the special sensory perceptive powers and their central correlation and integration in the brain. A clear sensorium conveys the presence of a reasonably accurate memory together with a correct orientation for time, place and person.

SENSORY HYPERACUITY. An unusual degree of sensitivity of any of the five senses.

SENSORY HYPNOANALYSIS. An experimental form of psychotherapy in which the patient focuses upon bodily sensations with or without verbal comment, which leads to an intensification of all sensory modalities. Visual imagery is greatly heightened by this process.

SENSORY HYPNOPLASTY. A technique in hypnoanalysis in which the hypnotized patient models clay to which various sensory stimuli have been added to stimulate basic primitive memories, associations, sensations, and conflicts. In sensory hypnoplasty, the multiple sensations are increased very markedly by changing the texture of the clay, its temperature, color, smell and consistency.

SLEEP LEARNING. The controversial theory that one can learn while asleep by means of a tape recorder and pillow speaker. See HYPNO-MNEMONICS.

SLEEP THERAPY. Usually refers to a prolonged drug-induced sleep for therapeutic purposes.

SOMATIC. Pertaining to the body.

SOMNAMBULISM. In hypnosis, a deep hypnotic state. Popularly, it refers to sleepwalking.

SOMNOLENCE. An oppressive drowsiness or inclination to sleep.

SOPHROLOGY. The area of medicine in which psychosomatic changes are deliberately produced in a controlled fashion, enabling clinical uses, elucidating psychophysiology and demonstrating the phenomena of psychosomatic behavior and their interrelationships in the interaction of psychological and organic factors. It includes the study of hypnotic phenomena, the study of relaxation techniques and Oriental systems of concentration such as yoga, Zen and its derivatives. See YOGA.

SPASTICITY. A marked hypertonicity or continual overcontraction of muscles, causing stiffness, awkwardness and motor incoordination.

STIMULUS GENERALIZATION. The spread of a conditioned response to some stimulus similar to, but not identical with, the conditioned stimulus.

STUPOR. A condition of lethargy and unresponsiveness with partial or complete unconsciousness.

SUBCONSCIOUS. Pertaining to mental activities of which the individual is not aware.

SUBLIMINAL PERCEPTION. Perception below the threshold of conscious awareness.

SUGGESTIBILITY. The capacity of an individual to be affected by such influences that may be called suggestions.

SUGGESTION. The process, especially indirect, by which mental processes in an individual or his behavior are altered by influence from without, in the absence of conscious volition on the part of the individual thus influenced.

SUGGESTION THERAPY. The use of waking or hypnotic suggestion in the cure or alleviation of disorders, particularly those of psychological origin.

SUPRALIMINAL. Above the threshold of consciousness.

SUSCEPTIBILITY. Suggestibility.

SYMPATHETIC DIVISION. A division of the autonomic nervous system that is active in emergency conditions of extreme cold, violent effort and emotions.

SYMPTOMATIC CURE. The removal of the overt symptoms of a disease without curing the disease itself.

SYNDROME. A group or pattern of symptoms that occur together in a disorder and represent the typical picture of the disorder.

TACTILE. Involving or referring to the sense of touch.

TIME DISTORTION. A hypnotic phenomenon whereby time is condensed or expanded in hypnosis.

TIME SENSE. A normal awareness of the passage of time.

TRANCE. Any of a number of differing psychological states characterized by temporary unawareness of the immediate environment or the suspension of normal voluntary activity.

TRANSFERENCE. The identification, usually unconscious, of some person in the individual's immediate environment with some important person in his past life. In therapy, the identification of the therapist with someone in the patient's past.

TRAUMATIC INSIGHT. A sudden awareness of previously repressed ideas disturbing to the patient.

TWILIGHT STATE. A state of disordered consciousness in which the individual performs purposeful acts for which he is later amnesic.

UNCONSCIOUS. That part of the mind or mental functioning, the content of which is only rarely subject to conscious awareness. A repository for data which has never been conscious (primary repression), or which may have become conscious briefly and was then repressed (secondary repression).

UNCONSCIOUS BODY IMAGE. See HALLUCINATED UNCONSCIOUS BODY IMAGE.

UNCONSCIOUS MOTIVATION. An incentive or drive that originates without conscious awareness.

VERIDICAL. Particularly indicates dreams that seem to correspond to events occurring at the time or later; prophetic dreams or visions.

WAKING HYPNOSIS. The state at which hypnotic effects are achieved without the use of the trance state.

WAKING SUGGESTION. A suggestion given in the normal state of consciousness that does not precipitate a waking state of hypnosis.

YOGA. A collective term for the various systems of mental and physical training designed to make the mind function at higher levels than normal.

YOGA or Y-STATE OF HYPNOSIS. According to Meares, the Yoga or Y-State of hypnosis is characterized by profound abstraction that is produced and maintained by an active effort of the will concentrated on a single idea. It differs from ordinary hypnosis in that the cerebration is active and controlled and concerned primarily with subjective ideation.

ZOIST. A journal published by Dr. John Elliotson, a British physician, in which he and others published their research findings on mesmerism.

References

CHAPTER 1

Arnold, M. On the mechanism of suggestion and hypnosis. *Journal of Abnormal & Social Psychology,* 1946, 41, 107-128.

Barber, T. Hypnosis as perceptual-cognitive restructuring: I. Analysis of concepts. *Journal of Clinical and Experimental Hypnosis,* 1957, 5, 147-162. (a)

Barber, T. Hypnosis as perceptual-cognitive restructuring: III. From somnambulism to autohypnosis. *Journal of Psychology,* 1957, 44, 299-304. (b)

Barber, T. Hypnosis as perceptual-cognitive restructuring: II. "Post"-hypnotic behavior. *Journal of Clinical and Experimental Hypnosis,* 1958, 6, 10-20. (a)

Barber, T. Hypnosis as perceptual-cognitive restructuring: IV. "Negative hallucinations." *Journal of Psychology,* 1958, 46, 187-201. (b)

Bartlett, E. A proposed definition of hypnosis with a theory of its mechanism of action. *American Journal of Clinical Hypnosis,* 1968, 11, 69-73.

Bellak, L. An ego-psychological theory of hypnosis. *International Journal of Psychoanalysis,* 1955, 36, 375-379.

Binet, A., and Féré, C. *Animal magnetism.* New York: Appleton-Century, 1888.

Brown, W. Hypnosis, suggestion and dissociation. *British Medical Journal,* June 14, 1919.

Burnett, C. Splitting the mind. *Psychological Monograph,* 1925, 34, (2).

Charcot, J. *Lectures on diseases of the nervous system.* London: New Sydenham Society, 1889.

Dorcus, R. Modification by suggestion of some vestibular and visual responses. *American Journal of Psychology,* 1937, 49, 82-87.

Elman, D. *Findings in hypnosis.* Clifton, N.J.: Dave Elman, Publisher, 1964.

Estabrooks, G. *Hypnotism.* New York: Dutton, 1943.

Eysenck, H. *Dimensions of personality.* London: Kegan Paul, 1947.

Ferenczi, S. *Sex in psychoanalysis*. (Translated by E. Jones). Boston: Richard G. Badger, 1916.

Freud, S. *Group psychology and the analysis of the ego*. New York: Liveright, 1922.

Gill, M., and Brenman, M. *Hypnosis and related states*. New York: International Universities Press, 1959.

Haley, J. An interactional explanation of hypnosis. *American Journal of Clinical Hypnosis*, 1958, 1, 41-57.

Heidenhain, R. *Hypnotism or animal magnetism*. London: Kegan Paul, Trench & Trubner, 1906.

Hilgard, E. Lawfulness within hypnotic phenomena. In G. Estabrooks (Ed.), *Hypnosis: Current problems*. New York: Harper & Row, 1962. Pp. 1-29.

Hull, C. *Hypnosis and suggestibility*. New York: Appleton-Century-Crofts, 1933.

Jacobson, E. *Progressive relaxation*. Chicago: University of Chicago Press, 1938.

Janet, P. *Major symptoms of hysteria*. New York: Macmillan, 1920.

Jones, E. *Papers on psychoanalysis*. London: Bailliere, Taindall & Cox, 1913.

Jones, E. The nature of auto-suggestion. *British Journal of Medical Psychology*, 1923, 3, 206-212.

Korth, L. *Curative hypnosis and relaxation*. Westport, Conn.: Associated Booksellers, 1958.

Kroger, W., and Freed, S. *Psychosomatic gynecology*. Glencoe, Ill.: Free Press, 1956.

Kubie, L., and Margolin, S. The process of hypnotism and the nature of the hypnotic state. *American Journal of Psychiatry*, 1944, 100, 611-622.

Lorand, S. Hypnotic suggestion: Its dynamics, indications, and limitations in the theory of neurosis. *Journal of Nervous & Mental Diseases*, 1941, 94, 64-75.

Lundholm, H. An experimental study of functional anesthesia as induced by suggestion in hypnosis. *Journal of Abnormal & Social Psychology*, 1928, 23, 338-355.

McDougall, W. *Outline of abnormal psychology*. New York: Scribner, 1926.

Meares, A. *A system of medical hypnosis*. Philadelphia: W. B. Saunders, 1960.

Mesmer, F. *Mémoire sur la Découverte du Magnetisme Animal*. Translated by V. Myers. London: Macdonald, 1948.

Muftic, M. A contribution to the psychokinetic theory of hypnotism. *British Journal of Medical Hypnotism*, 1959, 10, 24-30.

Pattie, F. The genuineness of hypnotically produced anesthesia of the skin. *American Journal of Psychology*, 1937, 49, 435-443.

Pavlov, I. *Experimental psychology.* New York: Philosophical Library, 1957.

Prince, M. *Clinical and experimental studies in personality.* Cambridge: Sci-Art, 1929.

Roberts, D. An electrophysiologic theory of hypnosis. *International Journal of Clinical and Experimental Hypnosis,* 1960, 8, 43-55.

Roberts, D. A proposed electrogenic process in hypnosis. *British Journal of Medical Hypnotism,* 1963, 15, (1), 2-10.

Rosenow, C. Meaningful behavior in hypnosis. *American Journal of Psychology,* 1928, 40, 205-235.

Salter, A. *What is hypnosis?* New York: Citadel Press, 1944.

Sarbin, T. Contributions to role-taking theory: I. Hypnotic behavior. *Psychological Review,* 1950, 57, 255-270.

Sarbin, T. Some evidence in support of the role-taking hypothesis in hypnosis. *International Journal of Clinical and Experimental Hypnosis,* 1963, 11, 98-103.

Schilder, P., and Kauders, O. *The nature of hypnosis.* (Translated by G. Corvin.) New York: International Universities Press, 1956.

Schneck, J. A theory of hypnosis. *International Journal of Clinical and Experimental Hypnosis,* 1953, 1, 16-17.

Shor, R. The three-factor theory of hypnosis as applied to the book-reading fantasy and to the concept of suggestion. *International Journal of Clinical and Experimental Hypnosis,* 1970, 13, 89-98.

Sidis, B. *The psychology of suggestion.* New York: Appleton-Century, 1910.

Skemp, R. Hypnosis and hypnotherapy considered as cybernetic processes. *British Journal of Clinical Hypnosis,* 1972, 3, 97-107.

Sparks, L. Quoted in Consciousness vs. unconsciousness in deep hypnosis. *Hypnosis Quarterly,* 1960, 6, (1), 36-46.

Teitelbaum, M. *Hypnosis induction techniques.* Springfield, Ill.: Charles C. Thomas, 1965.

Van Pelt, S. *Secrets of hypnotism.* Hollywood, Calif.: Wilshire Book Co., 1958.

Weber, W. A theory attempting to explain hypnotism. *Hypnosis Quarterly,* 1956, 2, (3), 28-32.

Weitzenhoffer, A. *Hypnotism: An objective study in suggestibility.* New York: John Wiley & Sons, 1953.

White, R. A preface to the theory of hypnotism. *Journal of Abnormal & Social Psychology,* 1941, 36, 477-505.

Wolberg, L. *Medical hypnosis.* Vol. I. *The principles of hypnotherapy.* New York: Grune & Stratton, 1948.

Wolpe, J. *Psychotherapy by reciprocal inhibition.* Palo Alto, Calif.: Stanford University Press, 1958.

Young, P. Experimental hypnotism: A review. *Psychological Bulletin,* 1941, 38, 92-104.

CHAPTER 2

Cooper, L., and Erickson, M. *Time distortion in hypnosis.* Baltimore: Williams and Wilkins, 1954.

Hartland, J. *Medical and dental hypnosis and its clinical applications.* Baltimore: Williams and Wilkins, 1966.

Wolberg, L. *Medical hypnosis.* Vol. I. *The principles of hypnotherapy.* New York: Grune & Stratton, 1948.

CHAPTER 4

Gindes, B. *New concepts of hypnosis.* London: George Allen & Unwin, 1953.

CHAPTER 5

Meares, A. Defenses against hypnosis. *British Journal of Medical Hypnotism,* 1954, 5, 26.

CHAPTER 6

Kroger, W. *Clinical and experimental hypnosis.* Philadelphia: Lippincott, 1963.

London, P. The induction of hypnosis. In J. Gordon (Ed.), *Handbook of clinical and experimental hypnosis.* New York: Macmillan, 1967.

Meares, A. *A system of medical hypnosis.* Philadelphia: W. B. Saunders, 1960.

CHAPTER 7

Ambrose, G. *Hypnotherapy with children.* London: Staples, 1961.

Elman, D. *Findings in hypnosis.* Clifton, N.J.: Author, 1964.

CHAPTER 8

Arons, H. *New master course in hypnotism.* Irvington, N.J.: Power Publishers, 1961.

Davis, L., and Husband, R. A study of hypnotic susceptibility in relation to personality traits. *Journal of Abnormal & Social Psychology,* 1931, 26, 175-182.

Hartman, B. *An outline of clinical hypnosis.* St. Louis, Mo.: The National Foundation for Research in Clinical Hypnosis, 1968.

Heron, W. *Clinical applications of suggestion and hypnosis.* Springfield, Ill.: Charles C. Thomas, 1957.

LeCron, L., and Bordeaux, J. *Hypnotism today.* New York: Grune & Stratton, 1947.

CHAPTER 9

Elman, D. *Findings in hypnosis.* Clifton, New Jersey: Author, 1964.

CHAPTER 10

Elman, D. *Findings in hypnosis.* Clifton, New Jersey: Author, 1964.

CHAPTER 11

Meares, A. *A system of medical hypnosis.* Philadelphia: W. B. Saunders, 1960.
Weitzenhoffer, A. *General techniques of hypnotism.* New York: Grune & Stratton, 1957.

CHAPTER 12

Baron, E. Hypnotic hibernation as therapy for certain emotional disturbances. *Hypnosis Quarterly,* 1958, 4, (2), 22-27.
Clement, P. *Hypnosis for therapists.* San Francisco: Author, 1970.
Coulton, D. Writing techniques in hypnotherapy. *American Journal of Clinical Hypnosis,* 1966, 8, 287-298.
Erickson, M. Pseudo-orientation in time as a hypnotherapeutic procedure. *Journal of Clinical and Experimental Hypnosis,* 1954, 2, 261-283.
Erickson, M. Indirect hypnotic therapy of an enuretic couple. *Journal of Clinical and Experimental Hypnosis,* 1954, 2, 171-174. (b)
Erickson, M. Special techniques of brief hypnotherapy. *Journal of Clinical and Experimental Hypnosis,* 1954, 2, 109-129.(c)
Erickson, M. Further techniques of hypnosis—utilization techniques. *American Journal of Clinical Hypnosis,* 1959, 2, 3-21.
Erickson, M. The use of symptoms as an integral part of hypnotherapy. *American Journal of Clinical Hypnosis,* 1965, 8, 57-65.
Gibbons, D., Kilbourne, L., Saunders, A., & Castles, C. The cognitive control of behavior: A comparison of systematic desensitization and hypnotically induced "directed experience" techniques. *American Journal of Clinical Hypnosis,* 1970, 12, 141-145.
Gibbons, D. Hyperempiria: A new trance state. Part II. *Hypnosis Quarterly,* 1972, 16, (3), 5-13. (a)
Gibbons, D., Hyperempiria: A new trance state. Part II. *Hypnosis Quarterly,* 1972, 16, (4), 8-16. (b)
Gibbons, D. *Beyond hypnosis: Explorations in hyperempiria.* South Orange, N.J.: Power Publishers, 1973.
Gibbons, D. Hyperempiria, a new "altered state of consciousness" induced by suggestion. *Perceptual and Motor Skills,* 1974, 39, 47-53.
Hartland, J. The value of "ego-strengthening" procedures prior to direct symptom-removal under hypnosis. *American Journal of Clinical Hypnosis,* 1965, 8, 89-93.
Hartland, J. Further observations on the use of "ego-strengthening" techniques. *American Journal of Clinical Hypnosis,* 1971, 14, 1-8.
Kline, M. (Ed.) *Hypnodynamic psychology.* New York: Julian Press, 1955.
Kroger, W. *Clinical and experimental hypnosis.* Philadelphia: Lippincott, 1963.

Kroger, W. Comprehensive management of obesity. *American Journal of Clinical Hypnosis,* 1970, 12, 165-176.

Kuriyama, K. Clinical applications of prolonged hypnosis in psychosomatic medicine. *American Journal of Clinical Hypnosis,* 1968, 11, 101-111.

Ludwig, A., Lyle, W., & Miller, J. Group hypnotherapy techniques with drug addicts. *International Journal of Clinical and Experimental Hypnosis,* 1964, 12, 53-66.

Moss, C. Brief successful psychotherapy of a chronic phobic reaction. *Journal of Abnormal & Social Psychology,* 1960, 60, 266-270.

Schneck, J. The psychotherapeutic use of hypnosis: Case illustrations of direct hypnotherapy. *International Journal of Clinical and Experimental Hypnosis,* 1970, 18, 15-24.

Walch, S. The red balloon technique of hypnotherapy: A clinical note. *International Journal of Clinical and Experimental Hypnosis,* 1976, 24, 10-12.

Wetterstrand, O. *Hypnotism and its application to practical medicine.* (Translated by H. Peterson.) New York: Putnam, 1902.

Wolberg, L. *Medical hypnosis.* Volume I. *The principles of hypnotherapy.* New York: Grune & Stratton, 1948.

Wolpe, J. The systematic desensitization treatment of neurosis. *Journal of Nervous and Mental Disease,* 1961, 132, 204-220.

Yanovski, A. Pseudo-orientation in time and anticipated parental death. *American Journal of Clinical Hypnosis,* 1972, 14, 156-166.

CHAPTER 13

Dengrove, E. A new letter-association technique. *Diseases of the Nervous System,* 1962, 23, 25-26.

Desoille, R. *The directed daydream.* New York: The Psychosynthesis Research Foundation, 1965.

Halpern, S. Hypnointrospection: Analytic and behavioral hypnotherapy. In M. Kline (Ed.), *Psychodynamics and hypnosis.* Springfield, Ill.: Charles C. Thomas, 1967, Pp. 71-145.

Hammer, M. The directed daydream technique. *Psychotherapy: Theory, Research and Practice,* 1967, 4, 173-181.

Kelly, G. Guided fantasy as a counseling technique with youth. *Journal of Counseling Psychology,* 1972, 19, 355-361.

Kretschmer, W. Meditative techniques in psychotherapy. In C. Tart (Ed.), *Altered states of consciousness.* New York: John Wiley & Sons, 1969.

Kubie, L. The use of hypnagogic reveries in the recovery of repressed amnesic data. *Bulletin of the Menninger Clinic,* 1943, 7, 172-182.

Leuner, H. *The use of initiated symbol projection in psychotherapy.* New York: The Psychosynthesis Research Foundation, 1966.

CHAPTER 14

Federn, P. *Ego psychology and the psychoses.* New York: Basic Books, 1952.

Fenichel, O. *The psychoanalytic theory of neurosis.* New York: W. W. Norton, 1945.

Freytag, F. *Hypnosis and the body image.* New York: Julian Press, 1961.

Freytag, F. The hallucinated unconscious body image. *American Journal of Clinical Hypnosis,* 1965, 7, 209-220.

Gindes, B. *New concepts of hypnosis.* London: George Allen and Unwin, 1953.

Hartman, B. Dreams and hypnoanalysis. *Journal of the American Institute of Hypnosis,* 1967, 8, (3), 27-29.

LeCron, L., and Bordeaux, J. *Hypnotism today.* New York: Grune & Stratton, 1947.

Meares, A. *A system of medical hypnosis.* Philadelphia: W. B. Saunders, 1960.

Meares, A. *Hypnography: A study in the therapeutic use of hypnotic painting.* Springfield, Ill.: Charles C. Thomas, 1957.

Muhl, A. Automatic writing and hypnosis. In L. LeCron (Ed.), *Experimental hypnosis.* New York: Citadel Press, 1965.

Raginsky, B. The sensory use of plasticine in hypnoanalysis. *International Journal of Clinical and Experimental Hypnosis,* 1961, 9, 233-247.

Rosen, H. *Hypnotherapy in clinical psychiatry.* New York: W. W. Norton, 1953.

Sacerdote, P., and Sacerdote, P. Some projective techniques in hypnotherapy: Induction of dreams and real versus hallucinated sensory hypnoplasty. *American Journal of Clinical Hypnosis,* 1969, 11, 253-264.

Schneck, J. *Principles and practice of hypnoanalysis.* Springfield, Ill.: Charles C. Thomas, 1965.

Stolzheise, R. Psychotherapy simplified. In L. LeCron (Ed.), *Techniques of hypnotherapy.* New York: Julian Press, 1953.

Watkins, J. Transference aspects of the hypnotic relationship. In M. Kline (Ed.), *Clinical correlations of experimental hypnosis.* Springfield, Ill.: Charles C. Thomas, 1963.

Watkins, J. Projective hypnoanalysis. In L. LeCron (Ed.), *Experimental hypnosis.* New York: Citadel Press, 1965.

Watkins, J. Hypnosis and consciousness from the viewpoint of existentialism. In M. Kline (Ed.), *Psychodynamics and Hypnosis.* Springfield, Ill.: Charles C. Thomas, 1967.

Watkins, J. The affect bridge: A hypnoanalytic technique. *International Journal of Clinical and Experimental Hypnosis,* 1971, 19, 21-27.

Wolberg, L. *Hypnoanalysis.* New York: Grune & Stratton, 1945.

Chapter 16

Hartland, J. The value of "ego-strengthening" procedures prior to direct symptom removal under hypnosis. *American Journal of Clinical Hypnosis,* 1965, 8, 89-93.

Hartland, J. Further observations on the use of "ego-strengthening" techniques. *American Journal of Clinical Hypnosis,* 1971, 14, 1-8.

Chapter 17

Cheek, D. Removal of subconscious resistance to hypnosis using ideomotor questioning techniques. *American Journal of Clinical Hypnosis,* 1960, 3, 103-107.

Cheek, D., and LeCron, L. *Clinical hypnotherapy.* New York: Grune & Stratton, 1968.

Denniston, P. A case for the ideomotor responses. *Journal of the American Institute of Hypnosis,* 1968, 9, (4), 15-19.

LeBaron, G. Ideomotor communication in confusional states and schizophrenia. *American Journal of Clinical Hypnosis,* 1964, 7, 42-54.

LeCron, L. A technique for uncovering unconscious material. *Journal of Clinical and Experimental Hypnosis,* 1954, 2, 76-79.

Shorr, J. *Psycho-imagination therapy.* New York: Intercontinental Medical Book Corporation, 1972.

Chapter 18

Hartland, J. *Medical and dental hypnosis and its clinical applications.* Baltimore: Williams & Wilkins, 1966.

Chapter 19

Boswell, L. The initial sensitizing event of emotional disorders. *Journal of the American Institute of Hypnosis,* 1961, 2, (1), 13-22.

Erickson, M. Naturalistic techniques of hypnosis. *American Journal of Clinical Hypnosis,* 1958, 1, 25-29.

Shorr, J. *Psycho-imagination therapy.* New York: Intercontinental Medical Book Corporation, 1972.

Chapter 20

Assagioli, R. *Psychosynthesis: A manual of principles and techniques.* New York: The Viking Press, 1971.

Gerard, R. *Psychosynthesis: A psychotherapy for the whole man.* New York: Psychosynthesis Research Foundation, 1964.

Gibbons, D. Hyperempira: A new trance state. Part II. *Hypnosis Quarterly,* 1972, 16, (4), 8-16.

James, M., and Jongeward, D. *Born to Win.* Menlo Park, Calif.: Addison-Wesley, 1971.

Chapter 21

Bryan, W., Jr. The walking zombie syndrome. *Journal of the American Institute of Hypnosis,* 1961, 2, (3), 10-18.

Bryan, W., Jr. *Religious aspects of hypnosis.* Springfield, Ill.: Charles C. Thomas, 1962.

Bryan, W., Jr. The Ponce de Leon syndrome. *Journal of the American Institute of Hypnosis,* 1964, 5, (1), 34-43.

Bryan, W., Jr., and Millikin, L. Injurious self-hypnosis induced while in church: Report of two cases. *Journal of the American Institute of Hypnosis,* 1962, 3, (2), 35-37.

Luria, A. *The nature of human conflicts: An objective study of disorganization and control of human behavior.* New York: Liveright Publishers, 1932.

Platonov, K. *The word as a physiological and therapeutic factor.* Moscow: Foreign Language Publishing House, 1959.

Van Dyke, P. Hypnosis in surgery. *Journal of the American Institute of Hypnosis,* 1967, 8, (1), 29-40.

Van Pelt, S. *Modern hypnotism: Key to the mind.* Westport, Conn.: Associated Booksellers, 1956.

Van Pelt, S. *Secrets of hypnotism.* Hollywood, Calif.: Wilshire Book Co., 1958.

Van Pelt, S. The dangers of stage hypnotism. *Journal of the American Institute of Hypnosis,* 1961, 2, (3), 28-33 & 49.

CHAPTER 22

Sullivan, H. *The interpersonal theory of psychiatry.* New York: W. W. Norton & Co., 1953.

CHAPTER 23

Bryan, W. J., Jr. The Ponce de Leon syndrome. *Journal of the American Institute of Hypnosis,* 1964, 5, (1), 34-43.

Bryan, W. J., Jr. Hypnosis and homosexuality. *Journal of the American Institute of Hypnosis,* 1967, 8, (1), 13-19.

Ellis, A. *Homosexuality: Its causes and cure.* New York: Lyle Stuart, 1965.

Fenichel, O. *The psychoanalytic theory of neurosis.* New York: W. W. Norton & Co., 1945.

Friedman, P. In S. Arieti (Ed.), *The American handbook of psychiatry.* New York: Basic Books, 1959.

Greenwald, H. Treatment of the psychopath. In H. Greenwald (Ed.), *Active psychotherapy.* New York: Atherton Press, 1967.

Guntrip, H. *Psychotherapy and religion.* New York: Harper & Brothers, 1957.

Hirschfield, M. *Sexual anomalies.* London: Francis Aldor, 1944.

Karpman, B. *The sexual offender and his offenses.* New York: Julian, 1954.

Kisker, G. *The disorganized personality.* New York: McGraw-Hill, 1964.

Kling, S. *Sexual behavior and the law.* New York: Bernard Geis Associates, 1965.

Levitsky, A. The constructive realistic fantasy. *American Journal of Clinical Hypnosis,* 1966, 9, 52-55.

Lindner, R. *Rebel without a cause: The story of a criminal psychopath.* New York: Grune & Stratton, 1944.

McGuire, R. and Vallance, M. Aversion therapy by electric shock: A simple technique. In C. Franks (Ed.), *Conditioning techniques in clinical practice and research.* New York: Springer, 1964.

Ritchie, G. G., Jr. The use of hypnosis in a case of exhibitionism. *Psychotherapy: Theory, Research and Practice,* 1968, 5, (1), 40-43.

Wolberg, L. *Hypnoanalysis.* New York: Grune & Stratton, 1945.

Wolberg, L. *Medical hypnosis.* Vol. I. New York: Grune & Stratton, 1948.

CHAPTER 24

Ludwig, A. *Treating the treatment failures.* New York: Grune & Stratton, 1971.

CHAPTER 25

Brown, T. Hypnosis in genitourinary diseases. *American Journal of Clinical Hypnosis,* 1959, 1, 165-168.

Bryan, W. The treatment of enuresis. *Journal of the American Institute of Hypnosis,* 1960, 1, (1), 35-39.

Cheek, D., and LeCron, L. *Clinical hypnotherapy.* New York: Grune & Stratton, 1968.

Collison, D. Hypnotherapy in the management of asthma. *American Journal of Clinical Hypnosis,* 1968, 11, 6-11.

Dunbar, F. *Emotions and bodily changes.* New York: Columbia University Press, 1938.

Gilbert, S. Juvenile enuresis: hypnotherapy in children. *British Journal of Medical Hypnotism,* 1957, 8, 43.

Hanley, F. Individualized hypnotherapy of asthma. *American Journal of Clinical Hypnosis,* 1974, 16, 275-279.

Hartland, J. *Medical and dental hypnosis and its clinical applications.* Baltimore: Williams and Wilkins, 1966.

Kisker, G. *The disorganized personality.* New York: McGraw-Hill, 1964.

Kline, M. (Ed.) *Hypnodynamic psychology.* New York: Julian Press, 1955.

Koster, S. Hypnosis in children as a method of curing enuresis and related conditions. *British Journal of Medical Hypnotism,* 1954, 5, 32.

Kroger, W. *Clinical and experimental hypnosis.* Philadelphia: Lippincott, 1963.

Leckie, F. Hypnotherapy in gynecological disorders. *International Journal of Clinical and Experimental Hypnosis,* 1964, 12, 121-146.
Maher-Loughnan, G. Hypnosis and autohypnosis for the treatment of asthma. *International Journal of Clinical and Experimental Hypnosis,* 1970, 18, 1-14.
Moorefield, C. The use of hypnosis and behavior therapy in asthma. *American Journal of Clinical Hypnosis,* 1971, 13, 162-168.
Rose, S. A general practitioner approach to the asthmatic patient. *American Journal of Clinical Hypnosis,* 1967, 10, 30-32.
Solovey, G., and Milechnin, A. Concerning the treatment of enuresis. *American Journal of Clinical Hypnosis,* 1959, 2, 22-30.
Van Pelt, S. J. An answer to asthma. *Journal of the American Institute of Hypnosis,* 1962, 3, (2), 7-12.

CHAPTER 26

Bryan, W., Jr. The treatment of alcoholism. *Journal of the American Institute of Hypnosis,* 1961, 2, (1), 38-50.
Kroger, W. The conditioned reflex treatment of alcoholism. *Journal of the American Medical Association,* 1942, 120, 714.
Kroger, W. *Clinical and experimental hypnosis.* Philadelphia: Lippincott, 1963.
Lemere, F. Psychotherapy of alcoholism. *Journal of the American Medical Association,* 1959, 171, 266-267.
Van Pelt, S. Alcoholics limited and hypnosis. *British Journal of Medical Hypnotism,* 1958, 9, (2).
Wolberg, L. *Medical hypnosis.* Vol. I: *Principles of hypnotherapy.* New York: Grune & Stratton, 1948.

CHAPTER 27

Ackerman, A. The T-group approach: Applications to a narcotic addict population. Paper presented at the California State Psychological Association convention, Coronado, Calif., January, 1971.
Ausubel, D. *Drug addiction: Physiological, psychological, and sociological aspects.* New York: Random House, 1964.
Baumann, F. Hypnosis and the adolescent drug abuser. *American Journal of Clinical Hypnosis,* 1970, 13, 17-21.
Bryan, W., Jr. Hypnosis and drug addiction. *Journal of the American Institute of Hypnosis,* 1967, 8, (3), 46-47.
Hartland, J. *Medical and dental hypnosis and its clinical applications,* Baltimore: Williams & Wilkins, 1966.
Kroger, W. *Clinical and experimental hypnosis.* Philadelphia: Lippincott, 1963.
Levine, J., and Ludwig, A. The hypnodelic treatment technique. *International Journal of Clinical and Experimental Hypnosis,* 1966, 14, 207-215.

Ludwig, A., Lyle, W., and Miller, J. Group hypnotherapy techniques with drug addicts. *International Journal of Clinical and Experimental Hypnosis*, 1964, 12, 53-66.

Ludwig, A., and Levine, J. A controlled comparison of five brief treatment techniques employing LSD, hypnosis, and psychotherapy. *American Journal of Psychotherapy*, 1965, 19, 417-435.

Truman, L. *Hypnotism may help cure girl of drug habit*. San Diego: Copley News Service, 1971.

CHAPTER 28

Hartland, J. The value of "ego-strengthening" procedures prior to direct symptom-removal under hypnosis. *American Journal of Clinical Hypnosis*, 1965, 8, 89-93.

Hartman, B. *The historical data questionnaire*. The National Foundation for Research in Clinical Hypnosis, 1971.

Ilovsky, J. Experiences with group hypnosis on schizophrenics. *Journal of Mental Science*, 1962, 108, 685-693.

LeCron, L. *How to stop smoking through self-hypnosis*. West Nyack, N.Y.: Parker Publishing Co., 1964.

Lieberman, L., Fisher, J., Thomas, R., and King, W. Use of tape recorded suggestions as an aid to probationary students. *American Journal of Clinical Hypnosis*, 1968, 11, 35-41.

Lindner, P. *Mind over platter*. Hollywood, Calif.: Wilshire Book Co., 1965.

Lindner, P., and Lindner, D. *Dr. Lindner's "Point System" weight control program*. Hollywood, Calif.: Wilshire Book Co., 1966.

Moreno, J., and Enneis, J. *Hypnodrama and psychodrama*. Beacon, N.Y.; Beacon House, 1950.

Peberdy, G. Hypnotic methods in group psychotherapy. *Journal of Mental Science*, 1960, 106, 1016-1020.

Salter, A. *Conditioned reflex therapy*. New York: Capricorn Books, 1961.

Serlin, F. Techniques for the use of hypnosis in group therapy. *American Journal of Clinical Hypnosis*, 1970, 12, 177-202.

von Dedenroth, T. The use of hypnosis with "tobaccomaniacs." *American Journal of Clinical Hypnosis*, 1964, 6, 326-331. (a)

von Dedenroth, T. Further help for the "tobaccomaniac." *American Journal of Clinical Hypnosis*, 1964, 6, 332-336. (b)

Wolpe, J. *Psychotherapy by reciprocal inhibition*. Stanford, Calif.: Stanford University Press, 1958.

Wolpe, J., and Lazarus, A. *Behavior therapy techniques*. London: Pergamon Press, 1966.

CHAPTER 29

Barber, T., and Glass, L. Significant factors in hypnotic behavior. *Journal of Abnormal and Social Psychology*, 1962, 64, 222-228.

Hilgard, E., Lauer, L., and Morgan, A. *Manual for Stanford profile scales of hypnotic susceptibility, forms I and II.* Palo Alto, Calif.: Consulting Psychologists Press, 1963.

London, P. *The children's hypnotic susceptibility scale.* Palo Alto, Calif.: Consulting Psychologists Press, 1962.

Shor, R., and Orne, E. *Harvard group scale of hypnotic susceptibility.* Palo Alto, Calif.: Consulting Psychologists Press, 1962.

Weitzenhoffer, A., and Hilgard, E. *Stanford hypnotic susceptibility scale, forms A and B.* Palo Alto, Calif.: Consulting Psychologists Press, 1959.

Weitzenhoffer, A., and Hilgard, E. *Stanford hypnotic susceptibility scale, form C.* Palo Alto, Calif.: Consulting Psychologists Press, 1962.

Weitzenhoffer, A., and Hilgard, E. *Stanford profile scales of hypnotic susceptibility, forms I and II.* Palo Alto, Calif.: Consulting Psychologists Press, 1963.

CHAPTER 30

Barron, F. An ego-strength scale which predicts response to psychotherapy. *Journal of Consulting Psychology,* 1953, 22, 327-333.

McNair, D., Loor, M., and Droppleman, L. *Profile of mood states.* San Diego, Calif.: Educational and Industrial Testing Service, 1971.

Verdier, P. *Conditioned response index.* Encino, Calif.: Tension Control Program, 1965.

Willoughby, R. Some properties of the Thurstone Personality Schedule and a suggested revision. *Journal of Social Psychology,* 1932, 3, 401.

Willoughby, R. Norms for the Clarke-Thurstone Inventory. *Journal of Social Psychology,* 1934, 5, 91.

Wolpe, J., and Lazarus, A. *Behavior therapy techniques.* New York: Pergamon Press, 1966.

CHAPTER 31

Goldstein, A. *Structured learning therapy: Toward a psychotherapy for the poor.* New York: Academic Press, 1973.

Index

317